The Essential Guide to Healthcare
Professional Wellness

Kristopher Michael Schroeder
Editor

The Essential Guide
to Healthcare Professional
Wellness

Proven Lessons from Leaders

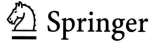 Springer

Editor
Kristopher Michael Schroeder
Department of Anesthesiology
University of Wisconsin
Madison, WI, USA

ISBN 978-3-031-36483-9   ISBN 978-3-031-36484-6   (eBook)
https://doi.org/10.1007/978-3-031-36484-6

This Springer imprint is published by the registered company Springer Nature Switzerland AG
The registered company address is: Gewerbestrasse 11, 6330 Cham, Switzerland

This book is dedicated to the love of my life who has stood by me through the years of training, long hours away from home, and absolutely outlandish ideas. She is the reason that I am able to stay well, a constant source of new adventure, and my hope for the future. I do not say it nearly enough, but I love you, I love you, I love you.

To my children, please know that you have been tremendous gifts and I apologize for the time spent away from you and the time that I have seemed distant while at home. I hope that the careers of your mother and I have shown you that there is a role for empathy and compassion in the world and that you feel free to chart your own path toward greatness.

Preface

Thank you.

Thank you for all that you have or are about to sacrifice on behalf of others. Thank you for the years of perseverance and dedication to a cause that so greatly benefits others and so greatly contributes to the betterment of society. Thank you for staying up late, waking up early, working weekends, working holidays, and never being able to give a straight answer about when you are going to be home at the end of the day. Thank you for going to work in the dark and returning home in the dark—spending only bookended vampiric time with your family. Thank you for missing too many milestones—first steps, first words, birthdays, weddings, and funerals—while effectively drifting apart from family and friends. Thank you for postponing life events (weddings, childbirth, house ownership, retirement) while you work to complete your training, pay back burdensome loans, or remain in a position out of obligation to your colleagues and your patients. Thank you for inventing reasons why Santa Clause visits your house on a different night than everyone else in the world on those Christmas days when you have needed to work. Thank you for coming home late, finding a bed full of kiddos that had tried to stay up long enough to see you, and choosing to either cram in or sleep in another room so as to not disturb the slumbering angels. Thank you for doing your job and doing it well while witnessing terrible tragedies—abuse, neglect, trauma, and loss—and absorbing these onslaughts to the soul without always having an outlet to share these events. Thank you for bearing witness to all this and, perhaps too often, keeping it to yourself so that your family doesn't lose faith in humanity. Thank you for doing all of this and more without the level of thanks that you deserve. Whether it is an administrative presence that fails to recognize the work and effort that goes into all that you do or patients/family/clients who fail to respect your efforts, please know that there are people in the world that see you, recognize your worth, and care about you and the work that you do.

Too often the work that we all do causes a stain on our lives that threatens to impede our ability to continue in our chosen profession. Like Lady Macbeth, too many of us possess stains or "spots" on our souls and consciences that too frequently prompt unsavory remedies (drugs, alcohol, infidelity, etc.). In fact, an insidious epidemic of burnout is plaguing healthcare and threatens more than just our happiness but the very lives of those tasked with caring for others. This epidemic seems functionally like an infectious disease that will indiscriminately infect those working in a variety of different fields. The problem with this epidemic is that it seems to only be increasing in scope and now represents a dire threat to our healthcare infrastructure. As a measure of the increasing scope and recognition of the burnout epidemic, a pubmed.gov search of "healthcare professional burnout" results in a logarithmic increase in publications over time with >1,600 burnout-related publications in 2021. As a specific example, an evaluation of a diverse group of critical care providers (physicians, nurses, respiratory therapists, pharmacists, and case managers) was published in 2021 and sought to further evaluate the impact of burnout in these providers in a "high stakes" environment [1]. Across all these groups, >70% experienced emotional exhaustion, 53% depersonalization, and 53% a lack of personal achievement. The authors of this study then divided the drivers of burnout into three core themes: patient factors, team dynamics, and hospital culture. Within these drivers, medically futile cases, difficult families, contagiousness of burnout, lack of respect between team members, the increasing burden of administrative/regulatory requirements at the cost of time with the patient, lack of recognition from hospital leadership, and technology all conspired to harm healthcare professionals and negatively impact their ability to care for patients and sustain meaningful careers. What simultaneously emerged from this study was that healthcare professionals are unaware of the degree of burnout symptoms that they are experiencing and substantially underreport their level of burnout. Healthcare workers experiencing burnout are caring for a wide range of patients and even those caring for infants are not immune to its effects. An observational study found that 46% of NICU nurses experience high levels and 37% moderate levels of emotional exhaustion [2]. Dentists, veterinarians, physical therapists, nurses, physicians, and healthcare professionals of all kinds are not immune to the effects of burnout, emotional exhaustion, and diminished career satisfaction. Recognition of these symptoms may be frequently reported in select professions, yet there are many professionals that suffer similar but underreported levels of burnout without the benefit of recognition. Nursing assistants, dental hygienists, and veterinary technicians are examples of careers where the plague of burnout is likely burning but the impact is, as of yet, unrecognized and underreported.

The impact of ignoring this situation might be tolerable to some, but a recent study suggests that a calamity is brewing that threatens our societies' ability to care for its sick and dying. A poll of 1,000 healthcare workers was completed in October 2021 during the COVID-19 pandemic. The results of this survey demonstrated that 18% of healthcare workers had quit their jobs during the pandemic and that an additional 31% had considered leaving. The cause of this exodus was ascribed to the pandemic, insufficient pay, burnout, and overall lack of opportunities [3]. Earlier pre-pandemic research had already suggested that nurses were electing to relocate or leave the profession in droves. In fact, a 2014 study reported that 17.5% of nurses leave their first job within 1 year and 33.5% leave within 2 years of starting a new career [4]. Those caring for our pets are impacted to an even greater degree with the average turnover for a veterinarian twice that of a physician and veterinary technicians experience turnover rates exceeding those of nurses [5]. Recent evidence suggests that the healthcare worker exodus may intensify as an increasing number of students are halting their training. As reported by the Nursing Standard in 2020, 33% of students pursuing nursing degrees are failing to complete their training and instead electing to pursue alternative career options [6].

The financial burden associated with seeking training to care for others is one that should certainly be considered among those contemplating a career in health-care. It is an unfortunate reality that the finances may not make sense for a variety of careers and students should enter these careers with their eyes wide open to the possibility of a lifetime of debt and the psychological burden associated with this constant yoke around their neck. Average student loan debt is only increasing and, while figures vary, can average $55,000 for nurses, $200,000 for physicians, $290,000 for dentists, and $180,000 for pharmacists. In 2020, the average veterinar-ian graduated with greater than $155,000 student-loan debt with a mean debt-to-income ratio of 2:1 [7]. These frequently insurmountable debt hurdles require that healthcare professionals either further prolong many of the milestones already accomplished by their peers (home ownership, marriage, childbirth, etc.) and/or make decisions that are based more on finances than personal preference (special-ization, job location, increased shifts, etc.). Beyond that, these financial obligations create significant stress, contribute to anxiety and may, in some cases, result in sui-cidal ideation or acts. It is no wonder that the Financial Independence, Retire Early (FIRE) movement has gained traction as more and more providers make decisions driven only to eliminate debt/accumulate wealth and, in so doing, potentially sacri-fice happiness and career longevity.

The mental health of healthcare professionals is constantly under assault. A 2014 survey found that nearly 1 in 10 veterinarians experienced serious psychological distress since graduation and that 24.5% of men and 36.7% of women reported depressive episodes [8]. A study of medical students found a 28% incidence of depression among medical students, while only 12.9% sought treatment for depres-sion symptoms [9]. Outside of the hospital and in the pre-hospital environment, ambulance personnel were found to have elevated levels of depression, anxiety, and posttraumatic stress symptoms and that the incidence of these findings was increased in those who were unmarried/no partner or with no access to peer support [10]. The COVID-19 pandemic amplified many of these mental health problems in healthcare workers. One study found that healthcare workers caring for COVID-19 patients were at elevated risk for severe moral distress, anxiety, depression symptoms, and mental disorders [11].

Collectively, we are at elevated risk for these mental health symptoms and, unfortunately, there are frequently barriers to seeking additional help. A lack of time to identify useful help can frequently represent a significant barrier in healthcare providers already working 60 h per week while attempting to be an engaged mem-ber of the family, social circles, and society. A lack of resources may be a barrier in some of the less lucrative medical specialties, and some work environments have not yet prioritized the care of their workers or are small enough to not have the means to supply these resources. There is also a stigma associated with mental ill-ness and mental illness therapeutics that may prevent some healthcare professionals from seeking the care that they need. Healthcare professionals are frequently accustomed to doing things on their own, pulling themselves up by their bootstraps, and acknowledging a need for help is not always second nature. However, an evaluation of the origin of the phrase "pull yourself up by your bootstraps" reveals that this was intended to reference a task that was impossible. As such, it is likely the case that there is a collective need to recognize that there is no shame in seeking assistance and those in leadership positions or benefiting from longevity-based stature should be more willing to model these behaviors.

The impact of sharing life with healthcare workers on families is one that is difficult to appropriately quantify. To a large extent, when one member of the family is a healthcare professional, the entire family takes on this occupation as their burden and something that must be managed. The end result of marital strife may ultimately be divorce, but the impact of a career in healthcare on the incidence of divorce does not provide a clear picture of the intricacies of these careers on family harmony. In fact, physicians have a rate of divorce (24.3%) that is significantly less than what is reported for non-healthcare professionals (35%). Women physicians seem to have a risk of divorce that is 1.5x their male counterparts and the etiology for this difference may be explained by traditional gender norms related to childcare and household management. Interestingly, as physicians work longer hours, their risk of divorce appears to decrease; physicians working greater than 60 h per week have an odds ratio for divorce that is 0.79 relative to their peers. Among healthcare professionals caring for humans, nurses have the highest rates of divorce (33%) compared to dentists (25.2%) and pharmacists (22.9%) [12]. For both female physicians and nurses, an additional theorized reason for elevated divorce rates in these groups is a power struggle that is fostered at home when a woman earns a higher salary relative to her male counterpart.

There is little data describing the impact of careers on the wellbeing of children when a parent is a member of the healthcare profession. However, it is clear that frequent sacrifices are made, and there is often a need or a perceived need to postpone starting a family. In addition, there is developing literature that suggests that those working in the healthcare setting suffer from a simultaneous onslaught of burnout symptoms and struggles with fertility. In one study, women physicians were found to have an increased frequency of time-to-pregnancy intervals longer than 1 year (18.4 vs 9.8%), suffered a higher rate of high-risk pregnancies (26.3 vs 16.3%), were more likely to seek infertility therapy (8.5 vs 3.4%), and experience a miscarriage (20.8 vs 14.6%) than members of the general population [13]. Another study demonstrated that women physicians suffered from infertility at a rate of 29.3% and that, in retrospect, 17.1% of those women would have chosen another medical specialty if they had known that it might have impacted their ability to conceive [14]. Similar struggles with pregnancy have also been found in nurses and appear to occur more frequently in nurses where heavy lifting was a normal work duty [15]. For many healthcare professionals, it is certainly accepted that biological, chemical, or physical exposures may impact a woman's ability to achieve or sustain pregnancy, but data is limited. From personal experience, I can relate to how struggles with infertility have now almost become an expected norm among healthcare professional colleagues and how the stress associated with this process can amplify already-existing problems with self-esteem and fulfilment. In our family, we struggled to conceive and suffered a miscarriage prior to the birth of our second child. Ultimately, it was only through a change in working conditions that baseline stress levels abated sufficiently for conception to then occur easily and without the assistance of medical adjuncts.

For a variety of reasons, multiple channels indicate that there is an increased risk of substance abuse and substance abuse-related mortality in healthcare professionals. Certainly, job-related stressors contribute to the increased risk in this population. However, it must be acknowledged that access to these agents certainly contributes to an increased risk in this group. Access to different anesthetic agents of varying potency in veterinary settings may further compound the problems associated with substance abuse. Further, the stigma of substance abuse and real or perceived risks of litigation or professional expulsion may contribute to hesitancy in seeking treatment for these types of disorders. Regardless, the impact of these substance abuse disorders on practitioners cannot be overstated. In fact, a study of anesthesiology residents found that the presence of a substance use disorder not only increased the risk of failure to complete residency or become board certified, but it is also increased the risk of adverse medical licensure actions and was associated with a 10-fold increase in post-residency mortality [16].

The culmination of these onslaughts is that healthcare workers are now taking their own lives in numbers that are staggering and unprecedented. Unfortunately, access to lethal means and understanding of physiologic processes may significantly influence the rate of attempts and success among healthcare professionals. Every healthcare professional is eventually touched by a colleague who chooses to end their own life. In most cases, we will all know of multiple colleagues who were so harmed by this profession that despite their atmospheric intellect were unable to visualize any future improvement in their situation. Those that we lose are often young and suicide represents the second-leading cause of death in those between the ages of 24 and 34. This tragic decision deprives parents of children and children of parents and leaves a lasting scar on those that are left behind. The impact of suicide on classmates, colleagues, and supervisors leaves a stain on entire programs that may never be removed and an impactful mark on all those who might even be seen as only tangentially connected to the person who took their own life.

Commonalities found among those who take their own lives include conflicts within a team, heavy workload, lack of autonomy, and work-family conflicts [17]. While much of the attention on suicide prevalence focuses on physicians, other healthcare service jobs such as dental assistants, massage therapists, and pharmacy aides experience rates of suicide that far exceed those of the general public and garner far less attention than received by their physician colleagues [18]. When physician suicide data is closely examined, the results are striking. Physicians are taking their own lives in staggering numbers and at a rate greater than 40% higher than the general population. Among physicians, anesthesiologists, psychiatrists, general practitioners, and general surgeons have been found to be at the highest risk of suicide [17]. Among healthcare professionals, those working in emergency departments, performing shift work, and those exposed to aggressive or violent patients appear to be at greatest risk of suicide [17]. Nurses appear to have elevated risks of suicide, but this rate of elevated risk remains an area in need of additional study. At greatest risk in the human medical community might be our most vulnerable and least well supported. A 2009 study found that the risk of suicidal ideation was high throughout medical school (6.6% of all students) but that it peaked during the fourth year (9.4% of students) as learners are compelled to pick a medical specialty and exposed to stressors associated with the residency match program [19]. This study reported additional concerning numbers for ethnic minorities who were found to have rates of suicidal ideation of 16.1% in trainees recognized as Indigenous, 13% in black/African American, and 7.6% in Hispanic trainees. Reasons for elevated risks of suicidal ideation in these groups are likely multifactorial but certainly diminished support and lack of faculty representation in these ethnic groups may be contributing factors. A 2014 survey found that veterinarians experienced suicidal ideation in 14.4% of men and 19.1% of women. Suicide attempts occurred in 1.1% of men and 1.4% of women and 400 veterinarians died by suicide between 1979 and 2015 at a rate more than 3.5x the general population [8, 20]. The organization Not One More Vet was created as an online support group for veterinarians around the world and now boasts more than 16,000 members. **If you are reading this now and are contemplating taking your own life or if you know of someone who is—please do not delay and contact the National Suicide Prevention Lifeline at 988 or 1-800-273-TALK (8255) or visit 988lifeline.org. In emergencies, dial 911.**

Despite this career dissatisfaction and risk of emotional and bodily harm, it is important to recall all that has been sacrificed and all that has been required to get to where you now are in your career. Throughout your education career, you have needed to fight to be near the top of the class and struggle to achieve high marks and distinguish yourself from your peers. I can imagine that many of you readers have been on this path since you were a small child, dressing up as a doctor, nurse, veterinarian, playing dentist to stuffed animals, or telling friends and family your lifetime career goals; those years of dedication may be contributing to the feelings of betrayal that you may now be feeling.

If all of this feels tragic and bleak—it is because it most certainly is. Sadly, if you are already working as a healthcare professional you are likely aware of the harmful effects of this profession on your own emotional wellbeing, your ability to interact with your family and your enthusiasm for remaining in your chosen profession. In addition, I can guarantee that you have witnessed first-hand the harmful impact of this profession on several colleagues. In the Lord of the Rings: The Fellowship of the Ring, Frodo proclaims that "I wish that it need not have happened in my time." To which Gandalf replies, "So do all who live to see such times, but that is not for them to decide. All we have to decide is what to do with the time that is given us." For far too long, we have accepted diminished mental health, suicides, substance abuse, etc. as standard operating procedure and a "cost of doing business" for those working in healthcare fields. However, it is likely time to now pressure administration and each other to take a more active role in the wellbeing of healthcare employees. We need a significant influx of resources to curb the pandemic of healthcare provider burnout and diminished wellness. What is needed is going to vary between organizations, but periodic assessments of healthcare employees need to be performed, and there need to be actionable items that emerge from areas identified as impacting the wellness of the professionals making the sacrifices to care for patients. It does nothing to recognize every year that the electronic medical record is causing harmful effects to healthcare professionals but then elect to do nothing about it. Action is required to assess these areas of harm and resources are required to implement solutions that will improve the quality of provider wellness and ultimately positively impact patient outcomes. Simultaneously, there is a great need to train and employ legions of mental health professionals that can be deployed to assist our colleagues with their mental health disorders, burnout, and potential desires to harm themselves. Through efforts to build support and resiliency into the system, society will benefit from a greater pool of qualified and well healthcare providers.

As healthcare professionals, we are accustomed to identifying a problem or arriving at a diagnosis and then working toward the development of a treatment plan. A 2018 article by Lia Novotny highlighted leading ways that healthcare professionals can increase fulfilment in their careers [21]. Connecting with patients, especially over the long term, seeing the impact that effective healthcare delivery can have on patients' lives, addressing social and behavioral determinants of health, developing rapport with clinical colleagues, tackling challenging cases, and maintaining scheduling autonomy and flexibility were identified as primary areas of emphasis in maintaining career satisfaction. While many of these areas exist within our collective sphere of daily influence, it may be challenging to envision pathways to achievement for the totality of the list. However, if your career satisfaction is low and (for example) autonomy and flexibility are currently outside the scope of what can be controlled, now may be the time to seek an alternate career opportunity that allows for an enhanced ability to influence and prioritize those things that are important to you.

If you are not yet working as a healthcare professional, this text is not intended to frighten you off. Providing healthcare is a blessing and a gift that can give your life significant meaning. From assisting in the process of bringing new life into the world to helping patients and their families embrace the process of dying and death, working as a healthcare professional represents one of the few career paths capable of leaving a lasting impression on people. People remember their OB nurse. People remember their surgeon. People remember the veterinarian who euthanized their pet. People remember the one phlebotomist who is always able to find their one vein. These interactions matter and make a difference in the world. In addition, this constantly changing environment represents an amazing opportunity for personal growth as you assimilate information and skills. Please come join us! We need quality, enthusiastic members to join our ranks and work with us to heal the world and the broken people in it. However, if you have not yet entered the healthcare community, now is the time to start building resiliency, start building strategies to maintain wellness, and build a community of friends and family to support you on your medical journey. You are going to need a team to get through this and what this team looks like—spouse, partner, parents, children, friends, close colleagues—is going to be different for everyone. The important thing to consider is building this team before the disaster, before the adverse event, or before the medical error so that they are in place and ready to be your support structure when you need it. And there is going to be a time when you will need it.

The intended audience of this book is as diverse as the perspectives on success and career fulfilment that are contained within. I have witnessed colleagues become disengaged, I have had colleagues take their own lives, I have had colleagues engage in substance abuse, I have witnessed faculty pour everything that they have into caring for patients to such an extent that their own health or their relationships with their families have suffered irreparable harm. At the same time, I have encountered faculty who seem to have managed to cultivate some mechanism to not only survive but thrive as a healthcare professional. These approaches to wellbeing seem to be as unique as the jobs that we all do, but the reason this book exists is to provide insight into tested and proven approaches to healthcare professional wellness. After reading this, my hope is that you can find some kernel of inspiration that turns the tide and makes a difference in your life and the lives of those important to you. If you have it all figured out already, please don't keep this information to yourself. Email me at happyinhealthcareproject@gmail.com and I will work to cultivate a collection of lessons from leaders that grows and evolves over time.

A quick note on how to read this book. This book is not necessarily intended to be read front-to-back, cover-to-cover. The lessons are grouped around broad topics—resiliency, bouncing back, family, spirituality, finances, and balance—with an introduction to the available literature followed by a number of lessons from your peers. As you progress through your career and encounter adversity, you may find one chapter that is more pertinent to you at that moment in time. You may also find that one lesson or a collection of lessons that just does not resonate with you. Great! However, with over 40 different perspectives, there are bound to be several authors where there is a connection and a kernel of inspiration that results in a positive change.

Thank you for all that you do!

References

1. Mehta AB, Lockhart S, Reed K, et. al. Drivers of burnout among critical care providers: a multicenter mixed-methods study. Chest. 2021; 161(5):1263-1274.
2. Thomas AO, Bakas T, Miller E, et. al. Burnout and turnover among NICU nurses. MCN Am J Matern Child Nurs. 2022; 47(1):33-39.
3. https://morningconsult.com/2021/10/04/health-care-workers-series-part-2-workforce. Accessed 1 Jun 2022.
4. Kovner CT, Brewer CS, Fetehi F, et. al. What does nurse turnover rate mean and what is the rate? Policy, Polit Nurs Pract. 2014;15(3-4): 64-71.
5. Salois M, Golab G. Are we in a veterinary workforce crisis? JAVMA news. 2021; Sep 15.
6. https://rcni.com/nursing-standard/newsroom/analysis/quitting-they-qualify-whats-behind-spike-nursing-students-dropping-out-177551. Accessed 1 Jun 2022.

7. Mattson K. Veterinary educational debt continues to rise. JAVMA news. 2020; Dec 3.
8. https://www.cdc.gov/mmwr/preview/mmwrhtml/mm6405a6.htm. Accessed 1 Jun 2022.
9. Puthran R, Zhang MWB, Tam WW. Prevalence of depression amongst medical students: a meta-analysis. Med Educ. 2016; 50(4): 456-468.
10. Reid BO, Naess-Pleym LE, Bakkelund KE, et al. A cross-sectional study of mental health-posttraumatic stress symptoms and post exposure changes in Norwegian ambulance personnel. Scandinavian journal of trauma, resuscitation and emergency medicine. 2022;30(1):1-9.
11. Spilg EG, Rushton CH, Phillips JL, et al. The new frontline: exploring the links between moral distress, moral resilience and mental health in healthcare workers during the COVID-19 pandemic. BMC Psychiatry. 2022. doi:10.1186/s12888-021-03637-w.
12. Ly DP, Seabury SA, Jena AB. Divorce among physicians and other healthcare professionals in the United States: analysis of census survey data. BMJ. 2015. doi:10.1136/bmj.h706
13. Gyorffy Z, Dweik D, Girasek E. Reproductive health and burn-out among female physicians: nationwide, representative study from Hungary. BMC Women's Health. 2014. doi:10.1186/1472-6874-14-121.
14. Stentz NC, Griffith KA, Perkins K, et al. Fertility and childbearing among American female physicians. J Womens Health. 2016; 25:1059-1065.
15. Gaskins AJ, Rich-Edwards JW, Lawson CC, et al. Work schedule and physical factors in relation to fecundity in nurses. Occupational and Environmental Medicine. 2015; 72:777-783.
16. Warner DO, Berge K, Sun H, et al. Risk and outcomes of substance abuse disorder among anesthesiology residents: a matched cohort analysis. Anesthesiology. 2015;123(4):929-936.
17. Duthell F, Aubert C, Pereira B, et al. Suicide among physicians and health-care workers: a systematic review and meta-analysis. Plos One. 2019. doi:10.1371/journal.pone.0226361.
18. www.cnn.com/2018/11/15/health/occupational-suicide-rate-cdc-study/index.html. Accessed 1 Jun 2022.
19. Goebert D, Thompson D, Takeshita J, et al. Depressive symptoms in medical students and resident: a multischool study. Acad Med. 2009; 84(2):236-241.
20. https://time.com/5670965/veterinarian-suicide-help. Accessed 1 Jun 2022.
21. Lia Novotny. 6 ways physicians find fulfilment in their work. Athenahealth.com. published November 29, 2018. Accessed 1 Jun 2022.

Contents

Part I

Balance

Abstract
For healthcare professionals, balance is vital to the maintenance of a successful career, relationships with others, and our own health. Without balance, there is an increased risk that healthcare professionals might view their career, not as a blessing and opportunity to help others, but as a significant source of stress, anxiety, and general unhappiness. The pathways to balance are as diverse as the work that each of us do. However, identifying a passion and external source of motivation can reflect back on and reinvigorate our passion for our careers. In addition, many of these activities can be associated with improvements in social support networks and physical, mental, and emotional well-being.

Keywords: Social support; Physical well-being: Mental health: Emotional health; Engagement; Coping mechanisms; Creative flow state

Thought Questions:
1. Beyond your career, what about you is unique? What about you represents something that others would recognize as interesting? How might you build upon those areas of interest to enhance your personal wellness?
2. List those activities/interests outside of work that bring you joy and help to define you and what you represent.
3. Consider interests from your past. Do you miss the presence of these activities in your life and is there a pathway to reincorporate these pursuits or find new ones?
4. How are you contributing to the betterment of the world? Given the personal benefits of volunteerism, are there opportunities for you to engage in these activities?

Become More Interesting

Kristopher Schroeder

Who are you? This question seems like it ought to be incredibly easy but how you answer might have a profound impact on your ability to maintain a meaningful career and a life in balance. If, without hesitation, you responded with your career designation as the answer to the "who are you?" question, maybe think a little bit deeper on what that might say about you, how that might devalue all the other components of what makes you truly unique, and what your response might say about how you value those around you. In our careers, as in all aspects of our lives, balance is key. Omit that crucial component and we risk burnout, we risk losing those we care about, and we risk having nothing left waiting for us at the end of our careers. Too often, healthcare professionals remain shackled to their careers into their 60's, 70's, and even 80's because they have not taken the time and prioritized achieving balance in their lives and cultivated a collection of people with whom to spend their time. When we prioritize work over everything else, it is at the expense of everything else. As Gary Keller pointed out, *"Work is a rubber ball. If you drop it, it will bounce back. The other four balls—family, health, friends, integrity—are made of glass. If you drop one of these, it will be irrevocably scuffed, nicked, perhaps even shattered"*(Keller 2012). Work is always going to be there. But, deprioritize these other components of your life and you risk achieving a solitary, unhealthy, and unhappy conclusion to your career.

"All work and no play makes Jack a dull boy. All work and no play makes Jack a mere toy" (Edgeworth 1825). In Stanley Kubrick's film *The Shining*, it became abundantly clear that too much of a devotion to a particular vocation introduces the potential for significant personal adversity. For healthcare professionals, the value of outside interests, hobbies, and passions are in many cases what makes us unique. These pursuits provide something to talk about, work for, and help make us relatable humans to the patients and clients that we care for. At some point, our careers will

K. Schroeder (✉)
University of Wisconsin School of Medicine and Public Health, Madison, WI, USA
e-mail: Kmschro1@wisc.edu

© The Author(s), under exclusive license to Springer Nature Switzerland AG 2023
K. M. Schroeder (ed.), *The Essential Guide to Healthcare Professional Wellness*,
https://doi.org/10.1007/978-3-031-36436-6_1

end, our children will leave the house, and life may seem less chaotic. Therefore, there needs to be something that still exists to give our lives purpose and stir a passion for participation in the world. What exactly that thing is that makes you look forward to the weekend or long to seek the clinic exits is going to vary between individuals, but there is a whole world of options to choose from.

It may be that you are blessed with an innate athletic ability that steers you toward an activity where you are able to achieve significant recognition. However, your achievement in a particular athletic endeavor really has little bearing on the happiness to be derived from involvement in that activity. Take running for example. Between 2008–2018, marathon participation increased 49.4%. Evaluating participation trends reveals that this growth in the field of running was not solely from individuals setting personal records (PR) or qualifying for the Boston marathon. In fact, it seems that those joining the ranks of marathon participants were of more mortal constitution and these runners were responsible for increasing the average marathon time by 3 min and 55 s over that same time period (Runrepeat.com 2022). These marathons have now become so popular that the largest race, the New York City Marathon, has 50,000 participants and a lottery is held to determine who might have the opportunity to participate. It has become simultaneously evident that it is never too late to start participating in these events. In fact, runners in the 40–49 year-old group are the largest segment of marathon participants. Even more inspiring is the fact that those in the 90–99 year-old category represent the fastest growing segment of the running community. From 2014–2017, this group's running participation increased 39% and serves to illustrate some of the inspiring things that can still be accomplished later in life (Forbes.com 2022). Too frequently, high-achieving healthcare professionals fall into the mindset of Ricky Bobby who, in the movie Talladega Nights: The Ballad of Ricky Bobby, was driven by the notion that *"If you ain't first, you're last."* Overcoming this mindset can be a difficult concept for many in the high-achieving sect, but there is significant opportunity for pleasure merely through participation. Read any posting from RunDisney events (everything from a 5 k to a full marathon) and you will encounter amazing and inspiring stories from those participants merely seeking to improve their health and enjoy participating in an event centered around a place that they love. The absolutely most inspiring stories come not from those who are seeking to win, PR, or qualify for another event but instead from those seeking to stay one step ahead of the balloon ladies (the balloon ladies represent a group of volunteers marking the slowest permissible pace). So, if you are the weakest competitor in the body building competition, if you are a slow enough swimmer that the lifeguards are considering asking you to stay in the kiddie pool, or if the only way that you can go for a bike ride is for the electronic bike to handle half the peddling—who the f#$% cares? Get out there!

A recent blog post presented several potential mechanisms by which involvement in sporting or fitness activities can improve overall wellness and help contribute to balance. For one, engagement in these activities can be a great opportunity to facilitate team bonding and the expansion of social support networks that might ultimately be important in the setting of future adversity. These activities can also be a tremendous opportunity for enhancements in employee engagement (Vantagefit.

com 2022). Nothing builds team unity better than rec league kickball and it is in these moments where bonds are built around insane commitments levied toward non-consequential athletic endeavors. These activities, even rec league kickball, can be a great way to achieve health and fitness goals. Ten-thousand steps is a great place to start but, in an era of increasing worship of our EMR overlords, significant time is now spent at workstations and any opportunity to get moving can pay substantial dividends. "Motion is lotion" and achieving the dream of a fit and active retirement is only possible if there is a steady commitment to fitness in the years leading up to retirement. Finally, engagement in athletics will inevitably lead to failure and micro-dosing with rec league failures enhances coping mechanisms for when a larger failure is encountered. The absolutely best baseball players in the world can only dream of a batting average of.400. As healthcare professionals, becoming comfortable with failure enhances our willingness to take chances and advance our fields. Without the freedom to make occasional mistakes, our collective professions would stagnate, and innovation would cease.

Exercise also has a number of important physiologic benefits that can benefit healthcare professionals. Decreases in stress, improved sleep, decreased fatigue, decreased illness-related work absences, improvements in mood, and a decreased incidence of depression and anxiety are all potential benefits associated with regular aerobic activity (Gerber et al. 2014; de Vries et al. 2015). Exercise may even make us better at our job through significant enhancements in brain health. It seems that exercise has the ability to improve cognition and concentration through a variety of mechanisms that can have immediate and long-lasting impacts. Exercise-induced increases in brain-derived neurotrophic factor (BDNF) have demonstrated the ability to increase neurogenesis, differentiation, proliferation, angiogenesis, neuroplasticity, neuron survival, grey matter volume, and cognition (Machado et al. 2015; Huang et al. 2014; Parry et al. 2018). With the constant acceleration of medical knowledge accumulation, it may become imperative to include regular aerobic exercise as a component of maintaining the ability to assimilate novel information and more effectively care for our patients. At some point, elevating exercise to the level of CME participation may be an effective mechanism for ensuring the longevity and fitness of our healthcare professionals.

It may be that our time spent outside need not be spent solely pursuing athletic endeavors to reap positive mental health benefits. Research is accumulating that demonstrates the positive impact of simply being/existing in nature and how spending time in that environment can provide a variety of physical and mental health benefits. Improved attention and cognition, decreased levels of stress, improved mood, improved sleep, a diminished risk of psychiatric disorders, increased levels of empathy, and improvements in cooperation have all been demonstrated through increased exposure to the natural world. Other studies have demonstrated that nature can provide an increase in happiness, subjective well-being, positive affect, positive social interaction, and be a source of purpose in life. There is emerging evidence that time spent in nature may have even more wide-ranging benefits and that it may be able to decrease systemic cortisol levels, alter prefrontal cortex blood flow, decrease blood pressure, improve immune function, and decrease the risk of obesity, cardiovascular disease, and diabetes. Nature exposure has even been reported to enhance the activity of natural killer cell activity and, through this activation, may have a role in enhancing the body's ability to eliminate cancer cells. There is some evidence to suggest that exposure to green spaces has the ability to even impact overall mortality—a benefit that many of our expensive pharmacologic therapeutics are often unable to replicate. The etiology for these positive effects is not entirely well known and they may simply be derived from decreases in stress via parasympathetic activation associated with immersion in the natural world. There is a biophilia hypothesis that suggests that humans have evolved to exist within the natural world and therefore have an innate need to occupy space in that environment. The attention restoration theory suggests that time spent in nature and disconnected may facilitate increased mindfulness through an enhanced ability to overcome mental fatigue and focus. Finally, it may be that exposure to chemicals emitted by plants (phytoncides) is responsible for some of the beneficial effects associated with exposure to nature (Jimenez et al. 2021; Li et al. 2007; APA.org 2022). Whatever the etiology of these nature-based therapeutics, it is difficult to conceive of a less expensive, lower risk intervention than spending a bit of time occupying space and reconnecting with the natural world. Consider this a challenge to seek out green spaces near you where you can engage all of your senses as you feel the warmth of the sun, smell the grass, listen to the birds, and watch the effect of the wind on the trees.

For many, the recognition and appreciation of beauty that is created not by nature, but instead by man, represents a significant path toward fulfillment and wellness. John Dewey provided a potential pathway for wellness through art appreciation when he wrote *"Art throws off the covers that hide the expressiveness of experienced things; it quickens us from the slackness of routine and enables us to forget ourselves by finding ourselves in the delight of experiencing the world about us in its varied qualities and forms. It intercepts every shade of expressiveness found in objects and orders them in a new experience of life"*(Dewey 1934). Art offers an opportunity to see and experience objects/activities/situations through a lens that can transform them into something that is more than their mere components. In art, there is an opportunity to identify beauty and promise, even in the shadow of horrifying tragedy. There is also an opportunity to appreciate an expression of grief, despair, and hopelessness and recognize the value associated with these powerful emotions. Through exposure to and appreciation of art, a variety of healthcare professionals have demonstrated the ability to enjoy enhanced wellness and satisfaction. A 2016 review provided evidence that the simple act of listening to music resulted in improved staff mood, efficiency, concentration, focus, energy, enthusiasm, positivity, and happiness. In addition, passive music listening was also demonstrated to decrease stress and tension while easing the process of caring for patients (Wilson et al. 2016). Indeed, a study of patients presenting for orthopedic surgery under spinal anesthesia found that the use of perioperative music resulted in patients with decreased self-reported anxiety and that these patients required fewer intraoperative sedative medications. Visual art displays in the workplace have also demonstrated the ability to provide substantial improvements in well-being through the creation of a better and more home-like work environment (Karpavičiūtė and Macijauskienė 2016).

While there certainly is an abundant amount of satisfaction to be derived from absorbing the creative works of others, there is evidence that engaging in the creative process may have substantial benefits for healthcare professionals themselves. In one study, nursing staff members engaged in silk painting activities once per week, outside of regular work hours, for a period of ten weeks (Karpavičiūtė and Macijauskienė 2016). Through engagement in these simple exercises, the nurses in this study were able to enjoy improvements in vitality/energy and their emotional wellbeing. In addition, participants in the limited-scale art project group reported decreased levels of general fatigue and barriers to activity. The authors of this study hypothesized that the beneficial impact associated with engagement in the arts may be related to entering a creative flow state. In this flow state, deep concentration and engagement may approximate what can be found through meditation and mindfulness and provide a link to the etiology of the improvements seen in mood and wellbeing. These activities may also produce beneficial outcomes through fostering a more positive work environment and thereby impacting a variety of wellness variables. Other collective healthcare setting art production activities have worked to combine collaboration, team-building, and environmental consciousness. In one example, a group of OR personnel worked to re-purpose otherwise discarded medication vial caps into large-scale art projects. This work brought together a variety of healthcare professional colleagues to create a lasting product that stands as a visual cue and reminder of their collaborative efforts and commitment to environmental sustainability (Zuegge et al. 2017).

Involvement in the arts may take many different forms. In one study, Irish healthcare workers were solicited to participate in a workplace choir (Moss and O'Donoghue 2020). This study demonstrated several qualitative benefits in healthcare professionals who elected to participate in this activity. Namely, they found that participation promoted social connection, enjoyment at work, and staff engagement. However, the authors did find that this activity had limitations in demographic appeal and, therefore, efforts would likely be needed to extend interest in this activity or alternate activities would need to be provided for workers uninterested in choir participation.

Clearly, exercise and other activities do not represent the only mechanisms through which healthcare professionals can develop a balanced and meaningful life. For many, leveraging their medical training as an opportunity to act in service to others and spread good in the world serves as a platform for wellness improvement. The perspective gained by individuals engaged in these activities is incredibly valuable and, in many cases, serves to place more petty concerns within a proper context. The benefits of these acts of volunteerism may not be entirely altruistic as there are well-documented physical, social, and psychological health benefits associated with serving others and focusing outside of the self. In a systematic review of studies evaluating the beneficial impacts of volunteerism for the volunteer, mental health appears to be significantly improved through altruistic acts. Through working on volunteer activities, decreased rates of depression and improved life satisfaction and wellbeing have been reported. In addition, previous research has demonstrated a 22% reduction in mortality in those engaged in volunteer activities (Jenkinson et al. 2013). Another study demonstrated that the impact of volunteer activities becomes more pronounced starting above the age of 40 and that these benefits continued to increase as the age of the volunteer increased (Tabassum et al. 2016). To a certain extent, it makes some conceptual sense that greater health benefits associated with volunteerism might be realized in older adults. Adults under the age of 40 are commonly engaged in childcare obligations, leaving fewer opportunities for additional activities. In addition, the care of these children represents a significant "purpose" for these individuals and serves as an effective antidote for generalizable malaise. Regardless, the results of these studies demonstrate the power of service and how those who routinely engage in service activities frequently seem to have a fount of wellness that can sustain them through various career difficulties. Consider how working to support and care for those in challenging conditions might change your perspective on the work that you do at your home institution and the value assigned to the resources made available to you there.

As written by Viktor Frankl in Man's Search for Meaning, *"Those who have a 'why' to live, can bear almost any 'how'"* (Frankl 1959). The challenge now is to discover a 'why' that exists outside of the sterile hospital or clinic environment. If significant time has passed since you last made an effort to engage in non-medical human activities, this may not be an incredibly simple task. However, micro-dose in failing. Try dancing. If it turns out that your dancing is so terrible that an ambulance is called for suspected seizure activity, maybe that isn't the best fit. Try something else. Keep trying something new until there is an activity/pursuit/passion that rises first to your lips when you are asked *"who are you?"*

References

APA.org. www.apa.org/monitor/2020/04/nurtured-nature. Accessed 1 Dec 2022.
de Vries JD, van Hooff ML, Geurts SA, et al. Efficacy of an exercise intervention for employees with work-related fatigue: study protocol of a two-arm randomized controlled trial. BMC Public Health. 2015:1117. https://doi.org/10.1186/s12889-015-2434-6.
Dewey J. Art as experience. New York, NY: A Wideview/Perigee Book; 1934.
Edgeworth, Maria. Harry and Lucy concluded. London England, R. Hunter, Baldwin, Cradock, and Joy, 1825.
Forbes.com. www.forbes.com/sites/robinseatonjefferson/2019/02/20/40-age-group-takes-lead-in-largest-marathon-study-of-recreational-runners-ever-conducted/?sh=7b7c7e166272. Accessed 01 Dec 2022.
Frankl V. Man's search for meaning. Boston, MA: Beacon Press; 1959.
Gerber M, Brand S, Herrmann C, et al. Increased objectively assessed vigorous-intensity exercise is associated with reduced stress, increased mental health and good objective and subjective sleep in young adults. Physiol Behav. 2014;135:17–24.
Huang T, Larsen KT, Ried-Larsen M, et al. The effects of physical activity and exercise on brain-derived neurotrophic factor in healthy humans: a review. Scand J Med Sci Sports. 2014;24:1–10.

Jenkinson CE, Dickens AP, Jones K, et al. Is volunteering a public health intervention? A systematic review and meta-analysis of the health and survival of volunteers. BMC Public Health. 2013;13:773. https://doi.org/10.1186/1471-2458-13-773.

Jimenez MP, NV DV, Elliot EG, et al. Associations between nature exposure and health: a review of the evidence. Int J Environ Res Public Health. 2021;18(9):4790.

Karpavičiūtė S, Macijauskienė J. The impact of arts activity on nursing staff Well-being: an intervention in the workplace. Int J Environ Res Public Health. 2016;13(4):435.

Keller G. The ONE thing: the surprisingly simple truth about extraordinary results. Austin, TX: Bard Press; 2012.

Li Q, Morimoto K, Nakadai A, et al. Forest bathing enhances human natural killer activity and expression of anti-cancer proteins. Int J Immunopathol Pharmacol. 2007;20(Suppl. 2):3–8.

Machado S, Paes F, Ferreira Rocha NB, et al. Neuroscience of exercise: association among neurobiological mechanisms and mental health. CNS Neurol Disord Drug Targets. 2015;14:1315–6.

Moss H, O'Donoghue J. An evaluation of workplace choir singing amongst health service staff in Ireland. Health Promot Int. 2020;35:527–34.

Parry DA, Oeppen RS, Amin MSA, et al. Could exercise improve mental health and cognitive skills for surgeons and other healthcare professionals? Br J Oral Maxillofac Surg. 2018;56:367–70.

Runrepeat.com. https://runrepeat.com/research-marathon-performance-across-nations. Accessed 01 Dec 2022.

Tabassum F, Mohan J, Smith P. Association of volunteering with mental Well-being: a life-course analysis of a national population-based longitudinal study in the UK. BMJ Open. 2016;6:e011327. https://doi.org/10.1136/bmjopen-2016-011327.

Vantagefit.com. www.vantagefit.io/blog/sports-and-wellness. Accessed 01 Dec 2022.

Wilson C, Bungay H, Munn-Giddings C, et al. Healthcare professionals' perceptions of the value and impact of the arts in healthcare settings: a critical review of the literature. Int J Nurs Stud. 2016;56:90–101.

Zuegge KL, Warren ME, Muldowney BL, et al. Promoting sustainable practices via art. Anesthesiology. 2017;127:206–7.

Running Club

2

Tonya M. Palermo

Early in my career, self-care and wellness behaviors were like old friends, always there when I needed them even if I didn't try hard to maintain regular contact. Running was an activity that I developed in college for exercise that I could choose to do when I had the time, and when there weren't other competing demands. I seemed to always find my way back to running without much effort.

My career as a clinician-scientist is demanding, with the challenges of maintaining federal grant funding, publishing papers, running a lab, and mentoring faculty and trainees. But the real challenge I learned after having three children was the difficulty meeting my own high expectations for my work productivity and for my role as a mother. My family grew exponentially and quickly in the span of a few years after having my first child and then twins. Self-care and wellness were not easily prioritized during this busy time as the mother of three children under the age of 3. For the first time in my life, I realized the intentionality that was needed for wellness. After having twins, getting back into running was a slow and painful process, pushing a double stroller around a hilly neighborhood in the early morning hours. It took many months to get out of basic survival mode and achieve any enjoyment or fulfillment from running.

Running has never been for the purpose of excelling at an activity – I have always been a mediocre runner. But, running is my centering activity, keeping me present-focused. I work out solutions, process my day, and figure out my thoughts and feelings. When life has been at its worst and most challenging, running breaks a cycle of negative emotions. Running also provides a nourishing dose of nature. Viewing the forest or the lake, feeling the mist on my forehead, sighting a deer or an eagle all provide an antidote to stress and helps restore my well-being. Running is a physical reminder that I can be fierce and face any challenge.

T. M. Palermo (✉)
University of Washington, Seattle, WA, USA
e-mail: tonya.palermo@seattlechildrens.org

As a new mother, the biggest impediment to my wellness was my sense of guilt and responsibility. After being away from my children all day to work, I struggled terribly with the idea of extending this time any further to do an activity for myself. I also struggled with the idea of ending work early to do an activity for myself. My guilt was so extreme I couldn't verbalize my desire to engage in self-care (through running) and couldn't ask for support. It just felt selfish. Practically, I also faced the very real barrier of encountering needy children upon entering the house. I made attempts to reclaim running – experimenting with having running gear in my car so that I could stop on my way home for a run if time permitted. I also attempted to run from work. These experiments had varying degrees of success, mostly because of my insurmountable guilt, which I found was not only present if I tried to run from home but also present if I tried to run from work.

In making a professional move to Seattle 12 years ago, I decided it was an opportunity to make changes to improve my self-care and wellness. I needed to reclaim my time from everything else trying to take it – to invest back into myself. I needed courage to identify my own needs as important and to prioritize them. My goal was to start my new position with a new approach to wellness. This was the birth of "Running club".

Running club has two main elements. First, it is a recurring appointment on my calendar on three workdays. This visible appointment is key for accountability to myself and to others who look and schedule on my calendar. In this way it has the same priority level as other meetings and events on my calendar. Second, Running club is a social activity, an event that I communicated to colleagues and mentees to encourage participation of others. To my delight, I had regular running partners over the years. This social connection further increased accountability but also enhanced the emotional benefits of running. It proved to be a wonderful way to role model wellness behaviors for my trainees (most of whom are women) who also needed an extra push to invest time in their personal well-being. Helping several women train for their first half-marathons and helping others get back into shape after childbirth were as rewarding as helping these same women write their first NIH grants.

Although many of my parenting responsibilities have changed as my children have grown into young adults and much of my work time more recently has been remote, Running club remains intact on my calendar. I have stayed true to the commitment and investment in my wellness. Running club is my symbol for maintaining a healthy lifestyle.

The Teller of Cautionary Tales

3

Steven L. Orebaugh

Life has offered me some interesting and unusual circumstances, and these have given me some unusual perspectives around which I could develop stories. I have been fortunate to have lived across the globe while growing up, completing my medical training, and during my early career in emergency medicine and later in anesthesiology. The U.S. Department of Defense was the driving force behind many of these moves. My father was in the Air Force- I was born in Japan and lived in a number of different towns, cities, and military bases until I was 12 years old, at which time we settled in central PA.

Early on in my medical training, I chose to pursue emergency medicine as a specialty, and I found that I had a strong interest in critical care medicine. After my EM residency and critical care medicine fellowship, I reported to the Navy to fulfill my obligation for the medical school scholarship that I had received. I spent the next 3 years on active duty at the Naval Hospital, San Diego, working as an emergency physician. Within a few days of reporting to officer training school in Newport, Rhode Island, Iraq attacked Kuwait, and the multi-national coalition, led by the United States, confronted Saddam Hussein. A few months later, I was sent overseas in support of the First Marine Division, as the triage officer in a small medical unit. Together with several other medical companies, we built and staffed a Marine Corps field hospital, a unique and challenging experience in the desert environment. There were numerous casualties when the ground war finally occurred, but fortunately the battles were quickly won, and the action came to a rapid conclusion. This diverse set of occurrences has served as an opportunity for me to pour my experiences into novels and memoirs that benefit from first-person knowledge and experiential encounters.

The evolving opioid crisis has touched my life several times – the current rate of opioid use and abuse has ensured that no citizen is immune to the impact of this

S. L. Orebaugh (✉)
University of Pittsburgh School of Medicine, Pittsburgh, PA, USA
e-mail: orebaughsl@anes.upmc.edu

deadly curse. The U.S. is in the throes of a true epidemic and opioid overdose is killing Americans in astonishing numbers. This is obvious each night on the evening newscasts. But very little attention is paid to the addiction that doctors, nurses, and other health care workers develop. By some estimates, as many as 15% of physicians, and a similar fraction of nurses, will develop chemical dependence. While much of this is due to alcohol, an increasing amount is related to opioids. Anesthesiologists and nurse anesthetists, who provide these drugs to patients daily, are among the most susceptible providers. Tragically, I have witnessed a number of ruined careers due to diversion and addiction among my peers and co-workers. I have also worked with residents whose lives have been irrevocably altered by these controlled substances. The allure of opioids is compelling, and once they are ingested or injected, a voracious appetite develops in the user, followed by destruction of health, profession, and relationships. I wrote "The Stairs on Billy Buck Hill" as a cautionary tale, one that may be able to influence those working in health care to avoid ever starting to use such drugs.

In the past, physicians and others in healthcare have been reluctant to admit our mistakes or reveal our imperfections. However, it is clear that hiding such things has adversely affected other professions. Given the destructive potential of opioid abuse in society at large, it is now imperative to address such shortcomings within our own ranks, in a transparent manner.

In this story, I found myself utilizing my own experiences as an anesthesiologist to flesh out the scenes, the action, and the characters. I have to admit that there is some of me in the protagonist, but I am fortunate that opioid use or abuse has never been a problem for me. It was a challenge to authentically depict how a physician who was in a position of great responsibility, with high self-regard, could somehow spiral into opioid abuse and even addiction, since he would be well-aware of the hazard that these drugs pose. Hopefully, I related a credible scenario, although at times I struggled to make it realistic.

I intended for the audience of the novel to be health care workers, and especially those who practice in acute care specialties, given their close proximity to opioids every working day. I thought it was especially important to alert trainees in these fields about the threat that opioids pose and reveal how vulnerable physicians and nurses are to the insidious influence of these drugs, especially if that first step is taken and principles are compromised.

I have spent the last 30 years involved in professional writing, to one extent or another, by virtue of being an academic physician. Our style of writing can be dry, quantitative, factual, and somewhat unrewarding. Or at least, unimaginative. There is some degree of creativity involved in trying to make such writing appealing and comprehensible to readers. But it doesn't allow for much in the way of soulful expression of the thoughts that emerge daily in all of us, about life, relationships, love, conflict, fulfillment, achievement. Part of me yearned to break free of the constrictive writing that I was doing for journals and presentations, and so I began to explore the right side of my brain (or maybe the left side? I'm left-handed!), through writing stories and novels.

Writing requires time, and like most people, I find that I don't have as much as I would like- I often stay up later than I should. The most favorable time for writing for me is during the quiet of evening, when I am best able to concentrate. I find inspiration in high quality writing in many different genres and have great appreciation for classic literature. Of course, I enjoy reading works by more recent authors as well. Last year, I read the Pulitzer Prize-winning "All the Light We Cannot See." This is truly impressive writing. My favorite authors include Conrad, Dickens, Hugo, and St.-Exupery. I'm impressed by their memorable characters, their careful plot development, and their delightful use of the language. It's important to have something to aspire to! I've read some of their books repeatedly, trying to understand how such renowned writers designed their characters and stories.

I am now entering the autumn of my career in anesthesiology. Within a few years, I expect that I will go to a part-time status, and hopefully can move to full retirement a few years later. It's essential, as one's professional life winds down, to keep the mind stimulated and engaged. I plan to do that in a variety of different ways as I move away from medicine. Writing, which is fun and fulfilling for me, will surely be an important part of that plan. If I am fortunate enough to have a book accepted for publication every few years, and if I can appeal to at least a small audience with each, that will be a great late-life accomplishment.

Taking care of patients is a great gift. I can't imagine having spent my life in any other pursuit. Creative writing, whether fiction or non-fiction, is very different. It allows me to share a part of myself with readers-if this captures their interest, and they approve, that is very satisfying.

Therapy Dog Life: Meet Reese Griffin

4

Jillian Rigert

My life revolves around my dog, Reese, and I am not ashamed to admit it. Reese is a cockapoo, a breed known for their empathy and affectionate personality. I met Reese when I was on survival mode, barely functioning and my clinic teammates told me – *"You should get a dog."* At the time, I thought – *"No way"*. I was in residency, lived alone, and my family was states away. I was struggling with grief on top of depression after my life had deviated off course as I was medically discharged from the military and had recently changed residencies. I had been overcome with loss of identities and the unexpected passings of young people close to me. I was exhausted in every aspect of life – Adding a puppy was clearly out of the question. Wasn't it?

Despite my reservations, *"just for fun",* I took a picture of a chocolate cockapoo that I found online, and I put the photo up in the residents' office *"for the future."* As I hung up the photo, I proclaimed, *"One day, I'd like to get a chocolate cockapoo pup like this and train him to be a therapy dog so that he can spread love and joy to the patients. I'll name him Reese, after the chocolate peanut butter cups."*

"He should be our clinic therapy dog. For us," laughed a clinic teammate. Sensing a strong element of truth and seriousness behind the chuckle, the idea stuck. As the week progressed, I kept checking on the puppy's availability online. Then, it happened—adopted—but not by me. While hopeful that the puppy had found a good home, my heart sank more than I had anticipated. In that moment, I turned my attention to the photo of the puppy's brother who looked much more timid. A sense of urgency overcame me. I immediately called to schedule a visit and placed a deposit before my doubts could take over.

When I met the pup, he held onto me tightly in a big embrace. The individual helping me meet Reese told me that I was the first person that this puppy had interacted with in this manner. He was so shy—just as his photo suggested, but I felt that we formed an immediate connection. In addition, I felt the support of a close

J. Rigert (✉)
Houston, TX, USA

friend who had passed a few years prior, reassuring me that this pup was the one I was supposed to meet. I named Reese in honor of my friend, and they share a middle name—Griffin.

When I brought Reese Griffin back to my apartment community, a family of dog lovers helped me raise him. This external support was much needed as a resident and first-time pup mom. With the approval of my clinic family, Reese came to clinic with me on many Fridays when we had literature review. Growing up in the medical clinic prepared him well for his future therapy dog visits. Reese and I became a certified therapy dog team, and thanks to COVID… he has been classically conditioned to join all Zoom calls (we did many virtual visits)… which makes professional meetings interesting at times. We also went in person to visit colleges and hospitals. At one of the hospital visits, we had one of the most memorable moments in my life when Reese visited a patient, and she said, *"You made this the best day ever. Thank you, Reese."* Tears of joy and gratitude for my pup filled my eyes and heart.

That moment was one I'd love to recreate as much as possible. When I think of the meaning I want to create from my life, I feel called to support people and walk with them as they navigate difficult times, diagnoses, and life transitions. I feel Reese was put into my life to share in the journey and teach me the way. Reese is full of life, love, and curiosity. He has helped me to get back into life so that I can live it to give it, and his unconditional love has helped me to see good in an often-dark world.

Reese taught me the power of community and has been my companion through major life and career transitions – never letting me feel alone. He acclimates well and taught me the importance of accepting help. Admittedly, I did interview 15 dog walkers before I was able to accept help, and I did change my job to minimize travel time and work closer to my companion. I see these decisions as a reflection of how Reese taught me to value time with loved ones and the importance of keeping our loved ones safe.

I share Reese with you – because I know he'd love to say hello and spread his love to you, too. May we all live life with puppy-like curiosity and harness this ability to spread more love and laughter. Please say hello if you see us on social media or in person as Reese loves attention and will make you an immediate BFF.

The Mirage of Arrival

5

Ketan Kulkarni

I was an A$^+$ student, academic ace, loved science, and was fascinated by mathematics. After high school, a difficult decision needed to be made. I wasn't going to be able to pursue all of math, physics, and biology. There were additional cultural considerations that factored into my ultimate decision to pursue a career in medicine. Being a doctor is often revered in Asian culture and is considered a very respectful and noble profession. Beyond the cultural considerations, I saw the ability to make a considerable difference and help someone in need of serious help as a calling that drew me toward medicine.

There were certainly a plethora of external influencers including personal, family, and societal expectations that might nudge someone to pursue a professional career in medicine. Such is the aura of this noble profession that the undecided or those desiring an opportunity to pursue a career as a physician even consult astrologists to predict their chances of success!! Thus, I decided to forego advanced studies in physics and mathematics, and the dream to become a doctor became a decisive goal. This decision is one that has had a long-lasting impact and it was not until 14 years after starting medical school that I landed on my first attending job. Despite, and perhaps because of the years that it took to get to this point, I remain dedicated to the delivery of excellent patient care, the pursuit of academic research, meaningful administration, and education.

In our society, physicians are often considered to be very successful, among the financially well off, set for life, earners of a high income, possessing a high net worth, members of the upper crust, the top 1% and so on and so forth!! They are often considered to be smart, hard-working, and compassionate people that place patients first (and rightly so)! Being a physician is often an aspirational career for millions across the globe and it is a true honor to be able to help fellow human beings in need of assistance and care.

K. Kulkarni (✉)
Dalhousie University, Halifax, NS, Canada

Despite all the benefits associated with a career in medicine, in 2017–2018 I found myself burnt out. I had a growing family, supportive spouse, my first permanent home, and a thriving career with a successful research and teaching reputation. I was climbing the academic ladder and earned my first promotion in only 5 years!!! However, the cost of this productivity was high. I was working at least 60–70 h per week or more, I was feeling tired all the time, and I found myself distressed and angry over what frequently were reasonably petty issues. I wasn't myself!! I was feeling that I wasn't enough!!

The etiology of my burnout was multifactorial but included practice limitations and a variety of administrative challenges including red tape, systems issues, and the inevitable politics of working in a group setting. In the midst of these challenges, I started wondering if the practice of medicine was fulfilling enough, in the long run, to justify my current feelings. I didn't see any obvious solutions, let alone easy ones. I tried to reach out to friends and colleagues and saw that the symptoms of burnout were etched across a wide group of professionals who had devoted their lives to caring for patients. Even renowned experts from all professions (regardless of their stage of career, their titles or their publication/speaking accolades) faced similar issues and were often burnt out. A very successful lawyer friend of mine who lives in a $four million mansion told me that he was the happiest when he had nothing. He had crammed 100-h work weeks most of his career and didn't know where it was all going. A lot of people, similar or different to this lawyer friend, were unhappy and it seemed as if this disease was only becoming more prevalent.

In an effort to address my symptoms, I sought answers in the repositories of medical knowledge. Unfortunately, literature searches in academic databases failed to yield answers to my questions or solutions to my condition. I attempted to engage colleagues in dialogue but found that many were wary to discuss out of concern for the stigma or the risk of being judged as weak or unfit. Many people said that those in our profession are expected to *"just put up with things"* and *"suck it up - maybe it will get better one day!"* Recognizing that I needed help, I sought mentorship from senior colleagues but found it to be only moderately helpful. I heard statements like *"medicine is not an office job, this is a calling not a profession, this work is 24/7/365, you are expected to comply, all academic work happens during after hours."*

Despite significant efforts on my part to seek solutions to my burnt-out symptomology, things got worse. Adding to my stress and feelings that there are just not enough hours in the day, my family continued to grow and generated additional responsibilities outside of work. At work, I faced more challenges and experienced the "short end of the stick" with politics. On more than one occasion, I found that my status as an ethnic minority resulted in standards being applied differently from those of other people in a particular organization. It was becoming extremely clear that I could not continue like this and that I really needed to figure out how to achieve balance and wellness! I was unfulfilled and unhappy despite being promoted, achieving international recognition for my academic accomplishments, earning a reasonable income, and enjoying the benefits of a caring and loving family.

As I sought a remedy for my condition, I realized slowly that I wasn't alone in this experience. A large majority of the public is often unaware that trainees dedicate more than a decade of their life to medical school and subspecialist training. These trainees frequently endure challenges in the course of their training. If one looks only at the time invested, medical students and other trainees can often approach 100-h work weeks. The concurrent accumulation of significant student debt frequently exceeds multiple 6 figures and saddles new graduates with what can seem like an insurmountable hurdle (Poon et al. 2022). Such dedicated training and work often requires people to place their passions and hobbies on the backburner and focus exclusively on their work. Oftentimes, the work of these early career faculty can be incredibly challenging as it extends outside of the clinical arena. Securing dedicated research/academic time or a long-term faculty or staff position becomes more challenging when one is trying to simultaneously build a clinical practice, perfect one's craft, and remain constantly connected to the influx of digital harassments. As Kulkarni et al. describe, the pressure to respond in a timely fashion to emails may evolve from a fear of missing out on educational, research or collaborative opportunities. There may also be fears that delaying a digital response might delay research projects or publications, complicate patient care, or disappoint a mentor or student. The result of tending to this "digital demon" before addressing the needs of the family and the self is a very poor work life balance! Often precipitating or exacerbating burnout! As careers progress and obligations and opportunities multiply, the "digital demon" only grows and can ultimately reach unsustainable proportions (Kulkarni et al. 2020; Kulkarni and Yoo 2022).

Ultimately, I came to reflect upon my own mortality and realized that my drive to establish my academic career had been at the expense of my external passions. I realized that those things that I once enjoyed were now a one and a half-decade old remote memory and that I needed to find a pathway to reconnect with those activities that once brought me joy. I simultaneously understood that I needed to achieve balance, acquire advanced leadership skills, focus on personal growth, find and connect with my tribe, and learn how to thrive and achieve fulfilment. No longer was it acceptable for me to only appear successful!!

I felt a clear need to expand beyond the traditional parameters of academic medicine. With the help of one of my core mentors, I started a 3-year longitudinal leadership training program. This career pivot challenged and revamped my thought process and understanding of what it meant to be successful. I also had the opportunity to sharpen my leadership, listening, and communication skills while working to obtain an executive leadership certificate. In the course of this self-improvement journey, I was exposed to the concept of life and career coaching. At the urging of my coach, I became a life coach and continue to actively engage in coaching other professionals to achieve high performance, success, and fulfilment. My focus is on SELF (Success, Entrepreneurship, Leadership, and Finance) (www.savvyphysician.ca).

In addition, I recognized that I needed to become well versed in finance (a skill lacking in many physicians). I practiced Do It Yourself investing for a few years before hiring and learning from a fiduciary finance advisor. I took control of the finances that were once controlling me through a variety of entrepreneurial pursuits including active and passive real estate investments. Now, I recognize the power that money can have and have over us. I have used my journey and understanding to advise friends, colleagues, and clients widely on the topic.

Finally, it was time to rekindle those outside interests that had been put on hold during medical training. In 2018–2019, I worked with a long-term friend to start an online art gallery. (www.atlanticfineart.com). In the course of pursuing this passion, I was afforded the opportunity to de-connect from medicine while meeting amazing collectors and making new friends. Now, when my work ignited an ember of burn out symptomology, I had an external passion that could extinguish the dread before it burned out of control.

Most certainly, I failed at several start-ups and small ventures. I made a lot of mistakes along the way and celebrate the fact that I have the opportunity to make new mistakes in the future. Each of these "failures" represent learning experiences that have made me better, made me stronger, and made me better equipped to help others as they struggle with their own journey.

This journey led to the creation of The Savvy Physician Facebook group (>1100 members today) - a group dedicated to addressing the common struggles of physicians through the creation of an online community dedicated to providing uplifting support. The main impetus of this group is to harness the collective experience of the tribe to help members get to the next phase more quickly, recognize more quickly those aspects of their life that might be holding them back or dragging them down, and work to identify pathways to improvement. In this journey, I have been fortunate to work with my friend Dr. Francis Yoo. As we worked together and deliberated on a range of topics and enduring questions, we wondered how is it that some people achieve incredible success across a range of measurable parameters? They are happy, deeply satisfied, live long, rich lives, enjoy positive emotions, cultivate relationships, undergo amazing spiritual journeys, and contribute to this world in meaningful ways, leaving a lasting and positive impact. This is observable, yet also so rare. *Why*? On the other hand, a large majority of people experience some form of distress or discomfort that dominates a significant portion of their life. This distress may be of such significance that it does not allow them to escape their fears and anxieties and can impact sleep, relationships, and increase the risk of substance abuse. Why do only some understand the meaning of life? Why do only some live to their full potential? Why do only some succeed, despite so many others doing difficult and smart work? What is it that determines what happens to us, our lived experience, our internal and external outcomes?

We could not find a resource that addressed these concerns in a simple and digestible format. Thus, we were compelled to present our investigations into these questions in our first book "The Legendary Quest"—a step-by-step approach that aims to guide the reader as they gain self-awareness and act as a catalyst in their own hero's journey of life. The appetite and reception for this book has been outstanding and has served as the catalyst for a second edition that is now in production—stay tuned!

With my ongoing personal growth and transformation, I now recognize that change and challenge are a part of life. I have experienced innumerable challenges along the way but am learning to manage them better and find the opportunities that may lay beneath, even if it's not immediately obvious. I now better recognize the common mental traps such as hedonic adaptation. We really do get used to any given situation over time, good or bad. Therefore, often a success or achievement feels great for some time but then no longer makes us happy, we get used to it or simply assume it. Another common trap is the "if then" hypothesis. How often do we say, *"if I achieve ...., then I'll be happy?"* Data is very clear that the achievement of a predetermined goal infrequently results in true contentment. With each accomplishment, there is always one more achievement, acknowledgement, shiny object that we hope will grant us the happiness that we are seeking. Unfortunately, those adapting this approach will find that all their work is never enough!! It's very common for academics to fall into the trap. Collectively, we need to cultivate an appreciation for how our work brings us happiness, all that we already have, all that we have achieved, and the greatness that we already possess. Comparing one's accolades or trinkets with someone else hardly matters!! If anything, its harmful. But it's easy to fall into that trap. Another key aspect is negativity bias...... negativity screams and positivity whispers. It's too easy and common for us to focus on negativity and ignore and minimize the positivity.

With my recently found awareness of myself and intentional behaviour, the burnout is long gone. I keep an eye on it when I feel challenged, when I experience failure, and when I'm overworked! I try to take that break when I feel like I need it. I recognize the mental traps sooner. I recognize the judging hyper-achiever in me trying to beat me down and learn to the tame him a little. While I still have many million miles to go, I feel that I am thriving!! I'm sure that if I can, you can too! But it's up to you!! Let's not fall prey to the arrival fallacy, the journey is at least as important as the destination!

I, Dr. Ketan Kulkarni, am a physician, a clinician-researcher, a passionate entrepreneur, an ardent advocate of financial literacy and independence with alternative income streams, an avid learner, a traveler, a photographer, an artist (and art enthusiast and antique collector) and a music buff.

I founded the Savvy Physician facebook group, co-founded thrive Rx course, and recently released my first book (The Legendary Quest). My podcast "The Legendary Quest Podcast" is available on apple, spotify, buzzsprout and more.

References

Ketan Kulkarni, Francis Yoo. The Legendary Quest, Published March 2022. https://www.amazon.com/Legendary-Quest-Professionals-Excellence-Fulfillment-ebook/dp/B09VBGPVSG.

Kulkarni K, Chiasakul T, Riva N, Eslick R. Casari C for the ISTH early career committee. Exciting times for the ISTH early career professionals. J Thromb Hemostat. 2020;18:2437–8. https://doi.org/10.1111/jth.15070.

Poon E, Bissonnette P, Sedighi S, MacNevin W, Kulkarni K. Improving financial literacy using the medical mini-MBA at a Canadian medical school. Cureus. 2022;14(6):e25595. https://doi.org/10.7759/cureus.25595.

The Correct Spelling of Wellness

6

Jalin Roberson

Medical School has been a rigid experience, always a straight line to prepare for the next task that needs to be completed. From studying daily for the next exam to working in a clinic to receive a good evaluation, medical school ultimately defines your day-to-day. Learning medicine does require this stringent path, but to me, it felt as though these walls were much too staunch and narrow, leaving no room for me to explore creativity and much less my wellness.

Memorizing the vast amount of medical knowledge we were being taught revived the saying I heard so often before starting medical school, *"it's like drinking from a fire hose."* That fire hose might as well have been physical with how much I felt its effect. Every day, the influx of new scientific terms and anatomical vocabulary flooded my brain, leaving me feeling more sunken than the day before. It became a repetitive cycle of feeling stressed over how much content was being taught, which turned into feelings of inadequacy due to not being able to absorb all the content.

Wave after wave of information, it felt as though I'd find myself crushed beneath medical education. There was no lightness to this instruction, with each new factoid seemingly growing in weight. I knew that I needed a way to combat this stress, pressure, and repetitiveness in some way that was healthy and cathartic. Even with those criteria decided, the search for such an activity was constrained by the limitations that medical school placed on my time.

I thought back to my childhood when I wrote raps and poems for my friends and family in elementary school. Thinking about the childish quips I used to pen down, I remembered how freeing and fun it was to just create for the sake of creation. I wanted to chase that freedom again, especially in the rigid path of medicine. I decided to write more for the sake of writing and as a protection against the burnout kindling within my mind.

J. Roberson (✉)
University of Wisconsin School of Medicine and Public Health, Madison, WI, USA
e-mail: jaroberson@wisc.edu

K. M. Schroeder (ed.), *The Essential Guide to Healthcare Professional Wellness*,
https://doi.org/10.1007/978-3-031-36484-6_6

Writing did not come back to me as quickly as I had hoped. It was awkward, a messy amalgamation of words splattered against the page as if a toddler babbled. I felt shame for wanting to restart. I felt shame in every pitiful poem I wrote. This shame shunned me from writing, from the creative wellness I sought. Even though my writing was clumsy, I continued with it. Eventually, I started to feel that same freedom I once felt. I did not magically get better. In fact, I'd hazard a guess to say I stayed the same as my elementary school self in my writing prowess. Letting go of the expectations of grandeur lifted a weight off my shoulders and allowed me to be happy, just letting out my emotions in the form of poems.

Halfway through my first year of medical school, the Covid-19 pandemic began, combining the difficulties of medical school with the isolation of the virus. Again, I felt overwhelmed, waking up day after day doing nothing but watching lectures and going back to sleep. I employed new tactics to take on this new challenge. I began writing while taking walks outdoors, sitting in the parks under shade, and on the edge of Lake Mendota. The rustle of the leaves and the turbulence of the water's surface were my company as my pen spilled my thoughts on paper. The isolation I once felt became a source of tranquility, a respite from the hustle and bustle of in-person activities and social obligations. I found comfort in the things that I could not change.

I transitioned from didactics to clinicals during the pandemic. My transition to clinical rotations was unique, as I moved back to my hometown of Milwaukee, Wisconsin to take part in the Training in Urban Medicine and Public Health MD track. Doing clinical rotations in Milwaukee and working closely with the underserved lit a fire under me and made me more excited to learn to become a physician. It also helped that my family still lived in Milwaukee and was always a 10-min drive away. Being able to see my family and our dogs whenever I wanted made the long clinical days easier to manage. I continued writing my poems, and they transformed into celebrations of hope. The change in scenery, being closer to my family and doing the type of medicine I always envisioned combatted the burnout I felt from didactics. Although the light at the end of the tunnel was far, I could now finally see it.

As I continued through medical school toward the finish line that was graduation, the heaviness of my future weighed on me. Sub-internships, STEP exams, and starting my application to residencies heightened the anxiety I harbored about my future. During this time, discussions with friends about their worries helped relieve my own. Commiserating in our collective misery during one of the most stressful periods in our lives became a source of wellness for all of us. We spoke about the hardships of applications, reviewed each other's personal statements, and gave positive affirmations to support one another. This was a different form of wellness, but made me realize how similar it was to the wellness I found in writing. The words of support my friends gave healed me in the same way as the thoughts I expelled in writing healed.

As my time in medical school draws to a close and I inch closer to my next chapter in the healthcare industry, I look back with fondness. Through all the trials and tribulations thrown my way during medical school, I somehow emerged on the other side in one piece. As I read again the musings of my experiences in medical school, I am content with how I perceived wellness to look like for me. The wellness that I cultivated and will take with me on my next step as a resident may not look the same as what wellness means to you. If I could leave you, the reader, with one sliver of advice, it'd be to seek the language of your unique wellness style early, because there is no correct spelling of wellness.

There and Back Again....

Kristin L. Long, Heather Gibson, and Mohammad J. Deen

For as long as I can remember, I have been fascinated by the world at large. Even as a young child, I felt compelled to learn as much as possible about other cultures. Dreams of "seeing the world" have long filled my mind, and not surprisingly, this love of adventure collided head-on with my love of science somewhere around 1995, when I sat, enamored, viewing the film "Outbreak." From that moment on, I dreamed of pursuing a career in medicine and hopefully working with hemorrhagic fever viruses in Africa. As they do, my dreams evolved throughout medical school, where I ultimately switched from an interest in pediatric infectious diseases into general surgery. I pursued my residency with plans to focus on pediatric surgery, guided once again serendipitously by multiple encounters with surgeons who spent a large portion of their careers living and operating across Africa. Recognizing that a career in surgery could be compatible with global health, and that these two together provided a unique opportunity for true adventure, I ultimately spent a month of my general surgery residency living in Kenya and working alongside local surgeons-in-training at Tenwek Hospital. This incredible experience laid the foundation for my current career in academic global surgery, and remains the part of my job that "gives" as much as it "takes."

I've spent a reasonable amount of time over the last few years researching surgical care in resource-poor settings and I developed an interest in wellness research before it was a particularly mainstream topic. In early February 2020, long before we knew what tragedy awaited the world with the impending COVID pandemic, I spoke at a medical mission conference about wellness, burnout, and

K. L. Long (✉) · M. J. Deen
University of Wisconsin School of Medicine and Public Health, Madison, WI, USA
e-mail: longk@surgery.wisc.edu

H. Gibson
Department of Surgical Oncology, MD Anderson Cancer Center, Houston, Texas, USA
e-mail: HMGibson@mdanderson.org

compassion fatigue, and how work in global surgery can, at times, be either the cause or the cure of these issues. Burnout, compassion fatigue, and as we've since learned, sustained emotional trauma from health care catastrophes, are pervasive in health care. The cumulative damage caused by the daily stresses of our jobs is severe. We bear witness to all manner of suffering in our patients, and sometimes in our colleagues, and must somehow muster strength to carry on and "get the work done." As we've learned in the last few years, any one of us can only take so much chronic accumulation of stress before we begin to break. Thinking of how routinely exhausting (physically, mentally, and emotionally) our work can be, many people have asked me how and why I choose to spend some of my much-needed time away performing surgeries in low-resource settings and how this could possibly be "refreshing."

Wellness speakers often espouse the benefits of things such as exercise, rest, mindfulness, time away, and other explicitly non-work-related efforts to mitigate things such as burnout. For me, I have found a huge component of my wellness within the work I am fortunate to do. No doubt that our day-to-day grind of healthcare here in the US can be frustrating at best, and is often demoralizing and full of inequity. In an endless cycle of mouse-clicks of the electronic medical record and bureaucracy of insurance and administration, I have found that one key to wellness and fulfillment for me lies in the "helping." Rendering aid to those in need was the core "WHY" of my desire to become a physician, and as many leadership experts have noted, the "how" we do a job we love may change dramatically but the "why" absolutely must remain central to our focus. The "why" equates with purpose.

My global surgery endeavors often find me in rural Western Kenya, working with Kenya Relief and a team of 15–20 other medical professionals, many from the US but increasingly more local Kenyan providers. Over the course of 4 clinical days, we complete a 1-day ambulatory preoperative clinic examining up to one hundred potential surgical patients, and then operating for 3 subsequent days on those identified as the most in-need and appropriate for surgery in this setting. My expertise is in thyroid surgery, and many of the patients we see have extreme examples of large, symptomatic goiters. Our surgical days often see each surgeon operating on 5–7 patients daily, with rapid turnover and long hours. Surgeons on our teams work with limited supplies and conserve resources meticulously, all the while ensuring top quality care and outcomes are provided to patients. Over 4 billion people in the world lack access to even the most basic surgical care and working to change this disparity is the most fulfilling part of my surgical career.

The days are long, but with each patient we operate on in this clinic, I am reminded of the reward of a job well done, and the internal fulfillment of challenging myself to find solutions to seemingly insurmountable challenges. There are heartbreaks, of course, as we often see disease states far beyond what can be cured or even treated and can feel helpless in the face of so much need. I am often reminded of one of my favorite quotes, from the Talmud, stating *"Do not be daunted by the enormity of the world's grief. Do justly now, love mercy now, walk humbly now. You are not obligated to complete the work, but neither are you free to abandon it."*

In addition, I have been privileged to share this experience with friends and trainees alike and have made many new connections along the way. The teams I have joined for these efforts have included many old friends, and I've never served on a team that didn't result in multiple new friends, united in purpose and working through adversity for the common good. Each individual patient I meet, each new colleague I work with, and each surgery performed provide personal connections that fill my spirit and keep me going….there and back again.

Working in Harmony

Heather Gibson

Ever since I was a young child, I have always wanted to pursue a career within the realm of science. I first dreamt of a career as a marine biologist, having a fascination with marine life. This developed into wanting to heal people, leading me into a career as a physician assistant. I was always interested in traveling and having new life experiences and wondered how I could use my skill set and knowledge to help on a global scale.

In my first few years of work, I was able to meet numerous health professionals that did global work and was finally convinced to travel to rural Western Kenya with an organization called Kenya Relief. At first it was overwhelming, and I was unsure of how I could actually make a difference with the insurmountable number of people that needed medical attention. Some cases were heartbreaking in that what they needed was far beyond the capability of the clinic in which we worked, but there were plenty of other patients that benefited greatly from the care provided by the team. With limited resources, it was a challenge to address all patients needs while conserving resources with the team. Even though the days were long and the number of patients needed to be seen never seemed to decrease, it still *"filled up my cup"* and provided me with a recharge that was needed for the daily grind back home. There were no multiple clicks, long documentation processes, and needing insurance pre-approval to get the job done, just people obtaining the care they needed, and a team of both local providers and visiting team members working in harmony to fully serve the patient.

A Promise…

Mohammad J. Deen

It was a promise to a total stranger made roughly 12 years ago. A promise to give back to those who have lost everything. A promise to help those who have nothing. This is my response when I am asked *"Why do you do what you do?"*. Roughly fifteen surgical/medical missions later, I still feel like I have yet to fulfill this promise. I truly can't recall the number of missions to be exact, just the stories. I don't recall the diseases, just the people. I struggled for some time post-mission because every place I go, I leave a piece of my soul there, and I always come back feeling a bit empty. I end up wanting to find this piece somewhere else, which is what leads me to my next destination, only to leave another piece wherever I end up.

Having done three missions in the harsh waters of the Mediterranean Sea as a medic on a rescue boat, I have encountered people who have fled a fast death via war, to potentially experiencing a slow death via the sea. You learn to appreciate life, and often, you learn to not take anything for granted. I have learned to live life through what I have seen. Through their eyes. To appreciate the small things. The smile. The hug. The greeting. The laugh. You learn to appreciate this over anything else because you realize these emotions are valuable and often these days, not felt so often. I witnessed these people show me these emotions despite everything they have been through, and this has really changed my mentality on life and how I go about my day. They have taught me much about life while they struggled to live, and for that, I am forever thankful. They left a piece of their soul within me, and I no longer feel as empty as I once felt.

Being an Environmental Steward in the Workplace

8

Michael L. Ma and Vivian Ip

For me, the definition of wellness is any aspect of my life which brings happiness, peace and balance. First and foremost to me is my family, our health and my career. These are all aspects which are directly impacted by my personal passion, environmental protection. Anyone who has been brought up with the formative and prominent 'ozone hole' news stories of the 90 s has always appreciated the concern of an ever-worsening environmental crisis. We cannot avoid daily reminders that these cornerstones to our wellness and happiness are directly impacted by climate change.

For my family, our best moments have always been outdoors. As a Canadian, we treasure all our seasonal exploits, watching our budding skiers snow-plow, getting that morning sunrise after a long hike, and our summers on the lake. We value our environment and the future it offers our children. Therefore, the warning of "Code Red for Humanity" issued last year sent a shiver down my spine. Climate scientists have been warning the world regarding global warming and the potential irreversible changes that could follow. Despite multiple warnings, many industries are still unregulated regarding carbon dioxide emissions and their effects on climate. One such industry is healthcare where our chosen profession contributes 10% of total greenhouse emissions in the US and 4% in Canadian healthcare systems.

At home, most of us recycle, compost and try to reduce the most wasteful aspects of day-to-day life such as plastic bags, plastic plates and all that endless packaging. However, home is only part of our life's picture. As physicians specializing in Anesthesia, we generate multiple times more carbon dioxide emissions at work than

M. L. Ma
Department of Anesthesiology and Pain Medicine, University of Alberta Hospital, Edmonton, AB, Canada

V. Ip (✉)
Department of Anesthesiology and Pain Medicine, University of Alberta Hospital, Edmonton, AB, Canada
e-mail: hip@ualberta.ca

K. M. Schroeder (ed.), *The Essential Guide to Healthcare Professional Wellness*, https://doi.org/10.1007/978-3-031-36484-6_8

the average person. This is because the volatile agents used in a general anesthetic are potent greenhouse gases. This means that in an average 7-h work day, the carbon dioxide emitted will be equivalent to driving from New York to west Ohio and this is practicing in an environmentally conscious way. However, despite the majority of Anesthetists choosing the more sustainable volatile agent, some may still choose a volatile agent that is more environmentally harmful. By choosing this less sustainable volatile agent, an average 7-h work day would be equivalent to having driven from New York to San Francisco three times! The most frustrating thing for me is that the choice does not impact patient care at all.

My career is a principal part of who I am. The ability to incorporate something so close to your heart, impact real change and make improvements through your job is, to me, the definition of fulfilment. As healthcare professionals, we attain a great level of achievement and gratification striving for improvement. Through colleagues and the literature, I am constantly learning about how my job affects the environment and I realize how much can be done. This process includes using safer techniques, instituting better systems, and always learning and educating others. Being environmental stewards in anesthesiology, we embody this via the use of sustainable techniques such as regional anesthesia and total intravenous anesthesia. These anesthetic options reduce the use of inhaled anesthetic agents. We have also instituted systems in our departments that highlight sustainable practice such as upgrading to more efficient anaesthetic machines and opting for reusable equipment whenever possible.

Not only do I practice in an environmentally sustainable way, I also find myself compelled to spread the message. Unfortunately, there are still many who are unaware of environmental sustainability in healthcare. It is important to seize opportunities to educate, as knowledge is the key to enabling change. Empowering others to do the right thing means we are closer to slowing down climate change and farther away from the 'irreversible line'!

"Green Anesthesia" has gained momentum as climate change has increased awareness. As a result, the academic community has accepted the importance of increasing education in this field. This has been evidenced by higher numbers of journal publications and international guest speakers dedicated to this cause. Environmental stewards have a great opportunity to educate on a much larger platform with the added benefit of increased leadership roles and responsibilities. In fact, through dedicated work with my colleagues I have had the honor of founding a special interest group within one of the largest anesthesia subspecialty societies, the American Society of Regional Anesthesia and Pain Medicine. From there, we also founded an Environmental Sustainability Section in the Canadian Anesthesia Society. One can gain a sense of peace, balance and fulfilment through engagement in environmental protection, improvements in medical practices for our greater society, and opportunities for simultaneous career progression.

Despite our best efforts, not everyone cares about the environment, and this can be quite disheartening. I am lucky to be surrounded by colleagues with similar values and aspirations. By working together and learning from each other, we have become good friends. Very often, when venting frustrations with this peer group, it can facilitate high levels of creativity. These conversations can sometimes lead to great ideas and projects to work on which boost morale. To have a group of friends in the workplace with whom you can relate to and confide in helps keep me vitalized. A social support element at work is crucial for us to thrive and stay focused.

Most notably I have seen how important this topic is for the younger generations of healthcare professionals. They are all too familiar with the concerns of greenhouse gas emissions leading to global warming and the threat to healthcare and humanity as a whole. It is a wonderful opportunity to connect with like-minded physicians over something so important to us all. It enables exchanges of new ideas and collaboration with a fresh perspective and I have hope that we are building the groundwork for future generations.

Green Anesthesia is still evolving and relatively novel with an ongoing need for exploration and innovation. Applying these principles in the workplace has permeated all aspects of my clinical practice and even extends beyond the boundaries of the hospital. As such, it has led to a further engagement and zest for what I do day to day. I feel a sense of contentment knowing that I am able to push past my comfort zone and contribute in any way I can to the advancement of this important mindset. The foundation we set now will continue to develop and progress well after my colleagues and I have all retired. This meaningful impact, I know will help me rest easy when I have left the clinical setting.

Ultimately, I feel passionately that through environmental protection in healthcare, one can find fulfilment as well as achievement. We are all too aware of how necessary it is for us to do our part, for our next generation and the generation after. Dedicating myself to this field has been a worthy cause in more ways than I can highlight. From implementing sustainable clinical practices and education to career advancement, it has provided balance and peace at work and beyond.

Part II

Family

Abstract

Each healthcare professional is generally blessed with an abundance of familial units. The traditional family unit is certainly forefront in the minds of most but the roles of this group can be assumed or supplanted by workplace of peer-group familial units. Whatever the case, it is important to consider the value provided by these individuals and take time to cultivate these relationships to maximize opportunities for connectivity and support. For the children and partners of healthcare professionals, it is critical to consider that these individuals share in the struggles encountered by healthcare professionals and their sacrifices should not be discounted. It must be acknowledged that healthcare professionals with children or who may become pregnant encounter bias in the workplace that may impact their career development. Finally, infertility is remarkably common and the impact of struggles with family planning may be a substantial source of stress for healthcare professionals.

Keywords: Infertility; Parenting; Childcare services; Breastfeeding; Divorce

Thought Questions:

1. If you have children, reflect upon some of the difficulties that you encountered with maternity/paternity leave or adequacy of time/space for breastfeeding. How might you make an impact within your organization to initiate change and improve conditions for the next generation of healthcare professionals?
2. Reflecting on your traditional family, are there additional opportunities to acknowledge and support this group that you might consider implementing? How has this group sacrificed to facilitate your ability to work as a healthcare professional?
3. Who in your workplace satisfies your definition of "family" and are there untapped opportunities to strengthen these relationships?
4. Utilizing an all-encompassing definition of family, how might you coordinate your life to spend additional time currency with this group and strengthen your social support network?

The Ties That Bind

9

Kristopher Schroeder

Family is not an important thing. It's everything.

–Michael J. Fox

"My family is my life, and everything else comes second as far as what's important to me.

–Michael Imperioli

This is my family. I found it all on my own. It's little, and broken, but still good. Yeah. Still good.

–Stitch

In each of our lives, no group of individuals produces similar levels of simultaneous support, stress, and irritation as those in our own families. To our credit, we generally acknowledge that these people occupy positions worthy of recognition for the value that they provide in our lives. However, no one is perfect and this group is frequently viewed as one that can be ignored or de-prioritized as we seek to further clinical or academic careers. However, it is important to recognize the role of these individuals, value their presence, and cultivate these relationships so that they are present and available when we find ourselves in a place of need. Beyond selfish needs, these individuals also warrant encouragement and support for the sacrifices that they have made and we must measure our careers to ensure our availability for these people.

K. Schroeder (✉)
University of Wisconsin School of Medicine and Public Health, Madison, WI, USA
e-mail: Kmschro1@wisc.edu

© The Author(s), under exclusive license to Springer Nature Switzerland AG 2023
K. M. Schroeder (ed.), *The Essential Guide to Healthcare Professional Wellness*,
https://doi.org/10.1007/978-3-031-36484-6_9

First, it is important to acknowledge that creating children can be incredibly difficult and is often a source of unseen pain for many of our colleagues. In one study of veterinarians, 17.5% of mothers reported at least one miscarriage and 17.6% required fertility treatments before ultimately conceiving (Wayne et al. 2020). In physicians, a study published in 2016 reported that nearly 25% have struggled with infertility (Stentz et al. 2016). Another study of women surgeons found that 42% reported a miscarriage and nearly half reported some pregnancy related complications (Rangel et al. 2021). Much of what leads to these difficulties in conception and healthy birth are unclear but delaying childbirth, stress, poor diet, long hours, lack of exercise, and potential workplace exposure may all represent contributing factors. While earlier childbirth is offered as a solution to this problem, fewer women who experienced childbirth during medical school reported an actively supportive workforce (68.2%) versus those who choose to have their children following training (88.6%) (Nytimes.com 2022). This all comes to little solace to those who deeply desire to start a family of their own and, despite Herculean efforts, are just not able to do so.

One of the mistakes far too commonly made is assuming that time spent with family and away from work will negatively impact our training and job performance. Attitudes regarding prioritization of family are tremendously pervasive in our profession and in many cases may discourage our trainees or early-career faculty from initiating family building or limiting the number of children they plan to conceive. In one study of general surgery residents, 42.5% of residents took fewer than 2 weeks of parental leave and many of these residents did not feel supported in their decision to even take leave of any duration. Of those who did take leave, 30.4% did not feel supported by other residents and 32.7% did not feel supported by faculty (Altieri et al. 2019). This is a problem that does not only impact the mothers of young children. A study of general surgery residency program directors revealed that 50% of programs provide only 1 week of paternity time and that these residents are restricted by poorly defined policies and the stigma associated with men taking this time with their newly born children (Castillo-Angeles et al. 2022). This simply does not need to be the case; our trainees and early-career faculty should be allowed the opportunity to cultivate relationships and care for new members of their families. Evidence demonstrating the ability to balance childcare responsibilities and medical training was provided by a study published in 2022. In this multicenter study, ophthalmology residents graduating between 2015 through 2019 were evaluated for the impact of parental leave on physician performance. In this study of 283 residents, 44 took a median of 4.5 weeks of parental leave. Importantly, this study demonstrated that those residents who took parental leave had no difference in research activity, ACGME milestone scores, or surgical procedure volume (Huh et al. 2022).

Unfortunately, the challenges facing new parents does not dissipate once our colleagues return to work. A 2019 study surveyed 413 residents in pediatrics, internal medicine, family medicine, and anesthesiology and found that 92% of mothers encountered difficulties with breastfeeding efforts following a return to work (Ames and Burrows 2019). In addition, 85% of these new mothers found that their mood was negatively impacted by the breastfeeding difficulties that they encountered at work. One interesting note in this study is that 40% of breastfeeding mothers worried that their pumping negatively impacted the team while only 10% of their co-residents felt the same. Similar findings have been found for medical students, attending physicians, and veterinarians (Wayne et al. 2020; Frolkis et al. 2020). Generally, the factors limiting successful opportunities to engage in pumping activities are inadequate and inaccessible space, time constraints, inflexible scheduling, and lack of colleague support. Even when children are no longer in their infant phase of life, too many mothers have been forced to endure long-lasting discrimination based on their parental status. In one study of veterinary mothers, 72.9% reported maternal discrimination and 58.4% reported at least one instance of workplace inequity based on their status as a mother (Wayne et al. 2020). In another questionnaire study of members of the Facebook Physician Moms Group, maternal discrimination was reported by over two thirds of the 947 respondents and this inequity limited opportunities for advancement, created a difficult work environment, and simultaneously disrupted efforts to create a sustainable work-life balance (Halley et al. 2018). It is easy to see how this "motherhood penalty" can foster feelings of stress, guilt, fear, and ultimately result in financial and career decisions with substantial and lasting implications. Beyond that, many of the study respondents reported that lack of support among colleagues frequently led to situations where the health of the mother had to be sacrificed to satisfy the unequal expectations of colleagues and leadership.

What then can be done about these problems that are too commonly encountered and perpetuated in our workplace? For one, we can normalize discussions of infertility to allow others to know that their struggles are common and have been encountered by countless others. Second, we can recognize that there are many of our colleagues suffering from the unseen pain associated with infertility and pregnancy loss. Finally, we can prioritize efforts to ensure that working parents are supported (via normalizing parental leave and providing an understanding and supportive environment that accommodates the needs of parents of young children) and not penalizing or stigmatizing these individuals because of their status as parents. Only these individuals can decide when they are in the correct season of life for them to assume leadership positions and they should not be denied these opportunities because of their status as parents.

The children of healthcare professionals may also be exposed to a variety of stressors that can have lasting and negative implications (Chesanow 1998). Early on, these children are often forced to come to the realization that the higher calling of their parents requires that they be relegated to second-class attention garnering status. Some healthcare professionals may also have difficulty transitioning from the dynamic that exists with patients to normal and functional familial interactions. Healthcare professionals may suffer from compassion fatigue with little emotional reservoir available to provide emotional support for their children. Finally, the children of healthcare professionals may be exposed to unrealistic and lofty academic and career expectations from their parents. When straight A's and upper 90th percentiles are the expectation and anything less is viewed as a failure, it can be difficult for some children to be seen as worthy or competent. Some of these difficulties are starting to change as society and healthcare professionals begin to recognize that there is an inherent value associated with creating boundaries and achieving some degree of balance. Ultimately, it is important to consider the impact of our careers on our children and consider how our behavior might impact their eventual well-being.

At this point, it is again critically important to acknowledge that there are many people who do not yet have children, do not want to have children, or who are unable to have children. For these people, you are certainly not bereft of family. For many, their spouse or partner represents the most intense family connection that they will come to experience. These relationships can be incredibly difficult to maintain when one of the pair works in the healthcare setting. Previous research into the arena of stressors encountered when one partner is a physician identified a number of potential pressures that seem to be impacted significantly by the gender of the physician. Both genders reported significant time pressure or that they felt that their careers allowed for insufficient time at home that negatively impacted their relationships with their spouses and children. Women physicians noted that they additionally had little time for themselves because they were also expected to shoulder an unequal share of domestic responsibilities. Men in this study expressed that night calls, on-call requirements, and the telephone were associated with significant interruptions to family life. Women physicians in this study frequently highlighted the challenges they encountered being a physician while also being asked to perform the duties of wife and mother. They pointed out that male physicians frequently benefited to a greater extent from a spouse at home tending to household responsibilities. Both genders felt that they suffered from a lack of support and that men expressed more frustration in not receiving support at home whereas women were more likely to experience stress from a lack of support at work. This same study evaluated stressors experienced by the spouses of these physicians and found that detachment, communication problems, concerns about their spouse's workload and interruptions represented the most common concerns (Rout 1996). In veterinarians, the impact of call shifts has also been found to be a significantly negative factor in the maintenance of intimate relationships and familial connections (Kohan et al. 2021).

Ultimately, the culmination of a relationship that cannot be salvaged is divorce. Divorce is not an uncommon occurrence in our society and general society rates of divorce seem to hover around 50%. Among healthcare professionals, nurses seem to suffer from the highest risk of divorce (33%), followed by dentists (25.2%) and physicians (24.3%) (Ly et al. 2015). For reasons that are unclear, the rate of divorce is significantly lower in healthcare professionals than the general population. Certainly, there are many reasons why healthcare professionals might find themselves in a relationship that is ending. Many of these reasons might be intimately tied to our collective professions and can include things like long and unpredictable hours, stress, and the same reasons why divorce remains incredibly prevalent in general society. If there are abuse or safety concerns, divorce represents an incredibly appropriate route. However, there are likely things that can be done to maintain and strengthen relationships that are struggling. First of all, there are marriage counseling professionals who are well-trained to speak with couples and help them navigate relationship difficulties. If there are large looming issues, strong consideration should be given to working with these people. Second, efforts to share your work experiences with your partner may provide tremendous benefit because it allows for a newly shared perspective on the challenges encountered in the workplace. In the course of our jobs, we have all witnessed horrible things. Abuse, assault, neglect, and the cruel fates that cause terrible things to happen to patients that are too young or seemingly undeserving of their medical diagnoses. These experiences have every right to impact you and your mood and it can be terribly difficult to leave these experiences within the confines of our work environments. Obviously, we are not able to speak in specifics about what we encounter at work. However, it does no good for our relationships for us to remain sullen and detached without providing a reason for the melancholy. Partners with careers outside of medicine have no concept of what is truly going on behind the walls of our hospitals and clinics. For most of us, we are not working in the world of Grey's Anatomy but our partners have no way of knowing what we are encountering if we are unwilling to open up about what struggles are occurring in the real world of healthcare. In addition, there does need to be some understanding of what those at home are going through. When we are constantly revising our estimated time of arrival, this has a huge impact on the wellbeing of those on the home front. These people are generally excited to see us, have frequently been waiting for longer than expected, and have often needed to upend their plans for the evening or weekend because of our inability to return home at a reasonable and predictable time. In these circumstances, it can be important to remain mindful of how difficult the endless waiting game can be for those at home and exercise compassion and patience if they are occasionally, and legitimately, annoyed.

Finally, we all need people in our lives and therefore should feel free to use the definition of "family" fairly loosely as we seek to fill our lives with those who can fulfill that role. Our work families can be a legitimate source of considerate and long-lasting support. The benefit of this family is that they have served with you on the front lines and share a number of work-related commonalities. In your pursuit of this work family, there can be benefits to seeking opportunities to make connections outside of your traditional profession-based silo. Gaining a diverse perspective from those that you work with allows you to consider additional viewpoints to situations and become a better team player.

References

Altieri MS, Salles A, Bevilacqua LA, et al. Perceptions of surgery residents about parental leave during training. JAMA Surg. 2019;154:952–8.

Ames EG, Burrows HL. Differing experiences with breastfeeding in residency between mothers and coresidents. Breastfeed Med. 2019;14(8):575–9.

Castillo-Angeles M, Smink DS, Rangel EL. Perspectives of general surgery program directors on paternity leave during surgical training. JAMA Surg. 2022;157:105–11.

Chesanow N. Think it's tough being a doctor? Try being a doctor's kid. Medical Economics. 1998;75(8):155–70.

Frolkis A, Michaud A, Nguyen KT, at al. Experiences of breast feeding at work for physicians, residents and medical students: a scoping review. BMJ Open. 2020;10(10):e039418. https://doi.org/10.1136/bmjopen-2020-039418.

Halley MC, Rustagi AS, Torres JS, et al. Physician mothers' experience of workplace discrimination: a qualitative analysis. BMJ. 2018;363:k4926. https://doi.org/10.1136/bmj.k4926.

Huh DD, Wang H, Fliotsos MH, et al. Association between parental leave and ophthalmology resident physician performance. JAMA Ophthalmic. 2022;140:1066–75.

Kohan L, Schoenfeld-Tacher R, Carney P, et al. On-call duties: the perceived impact on veterinarians' job satisfaction, well-being and personal relationships. Front. Vet. Sci. 2021;8:740852. https://doi.org/10.3389/fvets.2021.740852.

Ly DP, Seabury SA, Jena AB. Divorce among physicians and other healthcare professionals in the United States: analysis of census survey data. BMJ. 2015;350:h706. https://doi.org/10.1136/bmj.h706; PMID: 25694110.

Nytimes.com. https://www.nytimes.com/2021/09/13/health/women-doctors-infertility.html. Accessed 1 Dec 2022.

Rangel EL, Castillo-Angeles M, Easter ST, et al. Incidence of infertility and pregnancy complications in US female surgeons. JAMA Surg. 2021;156(10):905–15.

Rout U. Stress among general practitioners and their spouses: a qualitative study. Br J Gen Pract. 1996;46(404):157–60.

Stentz NC, Griffith KA, Perkins K, et al. Fertility and childbearing among American female physicians. J Womens Health. 2016;25:1059–65.

Wayne AS, Mueller MK, Rosenbaum M. Perceptions of maternal discrimination and pregnancy/postpartum experiences among veterinary mothers. Front Vet Sci. 2020;7:91. https://doi.org/10.3389/fvets.2020.00091.

Doctor Mom

10

Charlotte Grinberg

I can easily count the number of years since I graduated medical school: it's the age of my eldest child. I even missed my actual medical school graduation (very much disappointing my grandmother who always wanted to go to medical school herself) as I had already moved to establish prenatal care in the new city where I would give birth and start residency. Each time I welcomed my first three children to the world during residency and fellowship, our pediatrician would tell me: *"I could barely take care of myself during that time of my life. Why and how do you keep having children?"*

I cannot imagine being a doctor without being a mom, nor being a mom without being a doctor. These two intertwined identities have made me compassionately efficient and have been the foundation and guide for my adult life.

My ability to pivot between day and night-shifts, pull all-nighters, and take naps was developed by nursing and soothing my babies all hours of the day and night. My capacity to be patient with patients and their families was a learned skill taught by managing the simultaneous laughter, crying, and screaming of three kids under five. My colleagues have always been impressed by my organizational and multi-tasking skills, which for me is a constant state of mind. Whereas work can be the most draining time of the day for many, to me it often feels relaxing: I can use the bathroom or eat a meal without having three tiny humans stick their hands in the toilet bowl or grab my food right before it enters my mouth.

My experiences as a mother guide the compassion I try to always bring to the patient room. I am sensitive to the life logistics endured while navigating the health care system. Questions such as *"Who is taking care of your kids and for how long?"* and *"Do you need a breast pump? I can find you one in the hospital"* are intuitive. I care deeply about timely discharges and realistic follow-up. I can empathize with patients about how terrible it is to have explosive vomiting or diarrhea, or be so tired

C. Grinberg (✉)
Gilchrist, Hunt Valley, Maryland, USA

from sleepless days (chances are there was recently a stomach bug or respiratory illness traveling through my family). Usually I tell patients *"I can't even imagine"* when I see and hear what they are going through…but when it's a spouse or a child who is sick, I switch my language to share *"As a mother, I can only imagine how hard this must be."*

Motherhood also allows for the compassion I try to bring to myself. I know what it feels like not to expect or receive gratitude. No matter how many butts I've wiped, or sippy cups I've filled with the perfect ice:water ratio, a *"thank you"* is rare in my home. That's ok (except for my husband, he has to say thank you)--it was my choice to become a mom. It was my choice to be a doctor. People are sick, terrified, overwhelmed, and I don't need their appreciation to know I am doing a good job. Motherhood gives me strength in getting through the hard days at work. In medical school, I went to a lecture where a maternal fetal medicine specialist was talking about pregnancy and infant loss. Someone thoughtfully asked, *"how do you cope with it all?"* He described the feeling of hugging his own kids at the end of the day, how they managed to melt away the sadness and replace his heart with love. I know this feeling now, especially when I worked as an oncology hospitalist and I commonly saw young parents dying of metastatic cancer. A good hug helps. Too tired often to come up with original bedtime stories, I often share the stories of my patients (while honoring HIPAA compliance, don't worry) to connect my two worlds in my mind.

Motherhood has also guided and grounded me in career decisions. My family always comes first, which has been helpful in restricting geographically where to work; limiting my options helps avoid the paralysis of too many opportunities. I had a friend from medical school who applied to almost every residency program across the country because she could live anywhere. The financial and time burden associated with this application process was immense, and she ended up staying in the city she already lived in. I *saved* money during the residency application process, by subletting my apartment and staying with my in-laws while doing all my interviews in the one city where we had a lot of family. People always seem surprised that not only did I have children during my medical training, but I also published more than a dozen narrative articles. The secret to my writing is that it always took place in a delirious state before sunrise, after being woken up by one of my babies. I don't think I would have written as much without my children.

Although I try to maintain a positive attitude, there were challenges that needed to be overcome. It was hard to afford childcare during residency, and I tried to cut costs whenever I could. (Though, I regret biking during snowstorms instead of paying for parking). I put an inordinate amount of pressure on myself to exclusively breastfeed each child to make up for the feeling of not being physically present enough. I never advocated for more maternity leave past 7 weeks postpartum. I socialized less with coworkers outside of work. I still find that it's hard to be fully mentally present for patients and coworkers. There is that constant worry in my mind that I need to get home on time, that the school might call with a problem, the realization that we no longer have any fresh fruit in the fridge, and I have to run to the grocery store after a 12-h shift. It's easy to negatively compare myself to colleagues who don't have to always rush home, to feel jealous of their luxury of time.

Each person has their own desires and decisions, the things they can and cannot control, and their unique journey. My own process of becoming a mother was not an easy one. My childhood was full of unhappily married and then divorced patients, and I worried deeply if I would be able to provide my own children with love, stability, and empathy. My first pregnancy ended in a second-trimester loss, which convinced me for a period that I would never be able to have children.

In my work now as a hospice doctor, I meet patients daily in the final chapter of their lives. I listen every time for their wisdom and reflections on life. I've seen firsthand evidence that the cliche is true: in the end, it's all about family and community. You can tell who has lived a most full and kind life based on how many people surround their final bed. *"She was an amazing mom, sister, wife, and friend."* Photos on display everywhere. You can feel the warmth and gratitude and know this person's memory will live in the hearts of many. Much more rarely do you hear about people's professional careers. I'll never forget seeing a world-renowned author and artist who only had one visitor at the end of her life. She was divorced from her partner, estranged from both her sons. She died alone. These daily, drastically different experiences of bearing witness to the last chapter of life enable me to live in the present. It's fitting for my personality: I've always been someone who reads the last page of a book before the beginning.

Reflections

11

Melanie Donnelly

I have found myself spending quite a bit of time reflecting back on my life as my oldest enters his senior year of high school and my youngest his last year of middle school. I'm proud of the decisions my husband and I have made, and how we have provided our children with opportunities that continue to help them grow into the best version of themselves. It wasn't the easiest path to present, and I know at times it was an outright battle to get here.

From this moment, as I look back at the me of younger years, I find more language to help explain what was present, what was lacking, and what I can learn about myself by watching the younger me in action.

My baby B was welcomed into the world about 7 weeks prior to what we all expected. I had just started my first year of residency after a gen surg internship. The delivery was chaotic and I remember only bits and pieces of it. B was rushed off to the neonatal ICU after delivery where he spent his first 3 weeks of life. Part of that time on a ventilator and part of it learning how to feed and grow. I took time off and returned to my residency exhausted and barely ready to learn. B was still so little and there were still so many obstacles to him eating or breastfeeding and me learning how to use a breast pump. Inadequacy is the best way to describe how I felt for B's entire first year of life, both at home and at work. I was committed to feeding B breastmilk, especially given his difficult start to life. This required me to isolate on all breaks so I could pump. Interacting with fellow residents was a rarity outside of educational activities. At around 9 months of age, it was discovered that B had hydrocephalus and he had surgery....actually 2 surgeries a month apart. This was so disruptive to both my life and my training, and to my poor baby. I had no true idea what the implications of this would be for his life and I was worried for him. I was

M. Donnelly (✉)
Medical College of Wisconsin, Milwaukee, WI, USA

schoolhousemd.com, Hartland, USA

barely able to worry about me and how I was doing in my training program and really, I just tried to take it day by day and keep my head above water for the time being.

B began to thrive following his second shunt surgery and both he and I were headed onto a steady ladder of improvement. He received therapy to catch up on milestones, and I finally had a little bit of space to breathe, pause and study!!!

The most important resources for me during this time were my fellow mom residents. They understood my crazy thoughts and feelings, and we eventually formed a regular study group. We met in the wee hours of the morning while our kids were sleeping and the OR's weren't yet gearing up for the day. My program faculty exhibited super-human patience with me as well. This support was critical, and I can't overemphasize how important a supportive, caring, and honest program director was during this time. I understood when I was behind, and I also had all the belief I could improve and at least come close to catching up. That belief, in part, stemmed from the confidence my program director exhibited in my capability. What a gift!

I am dumbfounded when I consider how this young trainee managed to have this premature baby and successfully complete residency. All that on so little sleep....how? All that with so much less....how? All those difficulties and yet I recall that time as one the most cherished of my life ....

Maybe before she had the vocabulary or insight to verbalize it, she did know something about finding joy in the moment? Maybe she had grit before it was something we spoke about? And maybe she had the right support at the right time from the right people?

For now, I am doing my best to continue to find joy intentionally in my life each day. Connection to my kids, my spouse, my family, my friends...this feeds my soul and I continue to work on how to create more of this. Living in gratitude for me means appreciating the path that young woman, my former self, created for my life. It means appreciating the emphasis she placed on her baby B and the commitment she kept to become a doctor and complete training in order to craft the life I can live today.

I live my life today in hopes that my future self can reflect back someday and be proud of the path I choose now....

Your Family, Your Religion, and the Green Bay Packers

12

Kristopher Schroeder

In 1993, Jim Valvano delivered a speech at the 1993 ESPY awards that ought to be required viewing for anyone hoping to gain some perspective on life and how to prioritize the components in their life that truly matter. If you have not watched this speech, immediately—right now—put down this book and go to YouTube and search for "Jim's 1993 ESPY Speech." In this speech, Jim Valvano recounts a tale about how he, as a young coach, attempted to rally and inspire his Rutgers University freshman basketball team by compelling them to prioritize the various components of their life. The young coach Valvano sought to motivate his players by telling a story of how Vince Lombardi had previously motivated his players and assured them that they would be successful if they *"focused on three things above all else, your family, your religion and the Green Bay Packers."*

Indeed, family is recognized as vital to both a successful career and fulfilling life. How is it then, that these important people in our lives are too frequently relegated to the sidelines and that our career success or career failures can so easily overshadow those waiting for us at home? For me, my immediate nuclear family consists of my wife and three daughters. Throughout my career, what I have tried to keep in mind is that every missed event, every late night, and every time that work follows me home and significantly distracts me from the moments that I have with them, impacts these important people to the same degree that it does myself. What has occasionally been difficult for me to remember is that, in the eyes of my children, any academic title or accomplishment has tremendously little value or importance. Therefore, every decision that I make to improve my career or increase reimbursement has a cost and at some point, there becomes a need to sacrifice money, achievement, or recognition for time with family. I understand that my children are incredibly unlikely to recall any of my scientific publications or even exactly how many holidays that I missed, but what they will remember is how I spent my time with

K. Schroeder (✉)
University of Wisconsin School of Medicine and Public Health, Madison, WI, USA
e-mail: Kmschro1@wisc.edu

them and how I made them feel both when we were together and, unfortunately, when we needed to be apart.

Time is incredibly valuable and for that reason it is imperative to make the most of the time that you have with your family. At the same time, life is busy and children seem to have a way of getting involved in everything. I have made significant efforts to never make my children or the things that we do for them (athletics, lessons, etc.) a burden but instead an opportunity. The car rides that we have taken to various practices and events have provided us with amazing opportunities for them to recount to me what is important in their lives. Even in the 30 minutes before bed, a family routine of reading or watching a television show together provides an opportunity for daily connections. In your time together, it is important to celebrate the victories that emerge and understand that all victories don't need to be monumental to warrant celebration. Whether it is a high score or even good effort, use your time together to celebrate these accomplishments as a family and recognize that the success of anyone in the family is a reflection of the entire family unit.

As I have navigated my life and career journey, I have stumbled and at times neglected those at home in favor of my work family. In these times, I have recognized that it is important to make efforts to re-center and re-prioritize those within your sphere of family influence. For me, this has meant balancing career opportunities with the potential impact that they might have on my family. As a solution to this constant balancing act, you will find that my family is a constant companion with me at most academic meetings. At our large specialty meeting each October, my young children would frequently accompany me to the exhibit halls and they now recall this as an exciting opportunity to obtain some "unique" trick-or-treat gifts from exhibit hall vendors. At the conclusion of a lecture, I may see a triad of blond girls just outside the door of the conference room and am inspired to make a hasty retreat. Did I miss out on opportunities to collaborate and network? Certainly, but the time spent with my family on these trips is irreplicable and their opportunities to witness academic productivity has hopefully provided them with an understanding of why this work takes place.

My other familial stumbles have resulted from a poor ability to set boundaries between work and family life. To a certain extent, I see demonstrating a commitment to career and patients as a positive outcome and one that will hopefully resonate with the children. Where the inability to set boundaries can become more problematic is in the setting of work politics when these sorts of constant weights are carried around even after leaving the hospital. For me, it was only through disclosing these conflicts to my spouse and discussing these types of political insults that I was able to move past them and reach a place where I could appropriately dismiss harmful situations and individuals. Your spouse, significant other, or partner is truly something to be cherished and I have found it important to not overvalue the work that I am doing at the hospital while undervaluing any of the work that happens at home. My wife is remarkable in how she manages to tend to a flock of three children while working as a veterinary anesthesiologist. It has taken me a long time to get to the point where I am finally doing something that approximates my share of the work at home but it is incredibly important that I do this to demonstrate to the children the appropriate division of labor and to facilitate my wife's career by offloading home responsibilities.

I recognize that I am incredibly fortunate in the composition of my traditional family. I have an intact and supportive nuclear family and incredibly supportive and involved parents, sister, and in-laws. If this sort of traditional family support is not something that you have enjoyed, I do think that it is important to recognize that you are surrounded daily by a variety of work-based families and that these relationships can be cultivated to offer many of the same benefits as traditional families. In my place of work, I have a "family" of colleagues that I work with frequently and I often spend more time with them than I do my biological family. Within this work family, conflict is bound to arise but it is important to maintain these relationships and be available for each other in challenging times. In my immediate work group, I work closely enough with a group of four nurses that we share ownership of a pontoon boat. While I am not necessarily advocating for shared property ownership (this might ultimately end in catastrophic fashion), I am advocating for making important and lasting connections with your work colleagues. When a group of nurses that I worked with encountered a struggle with human resources regarding their compensation, you better believe that the entire group of physicians advocated loudly on their behalf. Cultivate these relationships and these situational "families" will be available for you in your time of need as well.

Finally, there are many who have unfortunately been a part of destructive or damaging family structures. I am incredibly sorry for this and I would challenge you to make certain that this cycle ends with you and that you make efforts to ensure that your children don't endure the same hardship that was a part of your upbringing.

In closing, I am certainly not perfect—far from it—and there are times that I have selfishly and foolishly prioritized career accolades and accomplishments over those that I work and live with. I am, however, inspired to become better and believe that there is an opportunity for nearly all of us to improve our ability to support the various families that we all have. I advocate now for you to again put the book down and search the internet for the Matthew McConaughey video—"Who's your hero." In this 2014 speech following an Oscar win for best actor, he describes his hero journey and how his best self is always 10 years in the future. In a similar fashion, my vision of myself as the best family member that I can be is me in 10 years. At that point, I will have learned to leave work at work and better respect the boundaries between the two, I will cherish all of the small victories that my children and spouse have and celebrate them appropriately, I will have ensured that my family is secure in the notion that they are loved and supported in all things and that they know that they have an unwavering advocate, and these families will not remember me as a physician but, instead, as a dad/husband/son/brother/co-worker that made them feel loved while remaining a casual fan of the Green Bay Packers.

Part III

Finances

Abstract

Money doesn't buy happiness. While that may be true, thoughtful financial planning is crucial to ensuring that the lack of enough money does not illicit unhappiness. While the scale of each of our financial enterprises and reimbursements may be varied, there are a variety of principles that should help to ensure that our personal finances remain in order and that we remain free to derive happiness out of working in our chosen professions. Ideally, we would all get to the point where we work because we choose to and not solely to earn a paycheck. While investments are certainly a key component of any successful financial management strategy, an equally important component is limiting expenditures and eliminating debt. Finance management can be challenging and there is often a taboo associated with the discussion of this topic. However, education and thoughtfulness are keys to understanding how your professional income can work for you and be utilized to accomplish your lifestyle and retirement goals.

Keywords: Personal finances; Financial literacy; Financial freedom; Debt elimination; Investing; Retirement

Thought Questions:
1. Do you have a plan for your finances and predetermined criteria for altering this plan? If you are unsure of any aspect of your current financial plan or investing strategy, do you know who to engage to understand how your hard-earned income is being managed?
2. Have you thought about your financial goals? When would you prefer to retire? Is there a time when you might prefer to reduce your employment percentage (work part-time)? How much money/revenue streams do you need to have accumulated to accomplish these goals?
3. Think about a financial mistake that you have made in the past. Are there looming financial decisions that might benefit from the experience that you have gained from a previous negative experience?

4. Are you strategically leveraging tax advantaged and employer contribution accounts to assist in the pursuit of a comfortable retirement? If you are unsure, do you know who you might be able to contact to gain assistance in this area?
5. Is there any chance that you might qualify for loan forgiveness? If so, are you completing all of the program requirements?

For Entertainment Purposes Only

13

Kristopher Schroeder

> *The host of this podcast is a practicing [physician, blogger, author, podcaster, etc.]. They are not a licensed accountant, attorney, or financial advisor. This podcast is for your entertainment and information only and should not be considered official personalized financial advice.*

A similar message greets each of us if we make it to the very end of any podcast that spends any portion of their time discussing how to best manage our personal finances and what strategies will be more likely than not to result in financial wellness. I have always found the need to include this disclosure statement somewhat amusing. Read a medical paper that might contain public health guidelines impacting the lives of thousands or even millions of patients and you will not find a similar disclosure that the information contained within is "for entertainment purposes only." Why is it that we have such an odd and bizarre relationship with money that we feel the need to frame conversations from content experts with disclosures? What is it about money that would make one feel so much more likely to seek retribution for a poor outcome? Money, finances, and our collective approach to this topic has become incredibly bizarre and the need to save is something that instead of being a blessing, may create significant anxiety and negatively impact mental wellness. What does seem increasingly clear is that the pathway to financial wellness is largely built upon a sustained commitment to thoughtful wealth building, restrictions in expenditures, and an understanding that there must be something that is sacrificed in order to accumulate wealth.

At one time, there really was little point to worrying about working more to accumulate significant financial resources. In a barter society, where goods and

K. Schroeder (✉)
University of Wisconsin School of Medicine and Public Health, Madison, WI, USA
e-mail: Kmschro1@wisc.edu

services are traded, there is a limit to how much material wealth can be obtained through hard work. Why do another surgery if I really don't need any more chickens? It was only after the invention of "money" or an abstract notion that some transportable and exchangeable item had an intrinsic value that could then be traded for goods/services, that there became an enhanced motivation to pursue a real accumulation of wealth. At the same time, it was only after the invention of money that a person would have the ability to engage in borrowing and the accumulation of significant debt. Clearly, much has changed since we first started accounts of debits and credits with rudimentary tally marks. Since we now generally live well beyond when we intend to stop working, there is a need to accumulate sufficient wealth to allow for continued survival (food, shelter, healthcare) and diversion (travel, entertainment) once there is no longer a reliable source of income.

While the notion of a plush retirement sounds amazing, early-career healthcare professionals frequently encounter hardships that are not well-recognized by the general public. The cost of education is now staggering and healthcare workers begin their careers with six-figure debt burdens that serve as shackles to a career that might ultimately/hopefully provide an opportunity to emerge from this mountain of debt. While statistics on career changes are difficult to interpret given that they are intertwined with job changes, the average member of the general public changes their place of employment nearly 12 times over the course of their lives (Edsurge. com 2022). Making a career change in healthcare frequently requires additional training time, additional debt accumulation, and additional lost potential income. Even seeking one additional year of specialty or subspecialty training might ultimately result in the loss of hundreds of thousands of dollars (Whitecoatinvestor. com 2022). When healthcare professionals finally begin their careers and start paying off education debt in their 30's, they do so while frequently not having yet contributed to retirement accounts and find themselves well-behind their peers who have been doing so for what may be over a decade.

When one works in exchange for money, what they are generally doing is exchanging increments of their life for financial reimbursement. How much of your life are you willing to sacrifice in exchange for the currency of the realm and how much money is required to buy your time away from your family, your interests, and your time away from clinical medicine? If we engage in a simple exercise that better demonstrates the sacrifices that we are making in exchange for our salaries, one place to look is at the amount of time committed to our profession. In each week, there are 168 h. If we sleep 8 h a night, that leaves 112 waking hours for us to use as we see fit. A 40-h work week gets you to over 35% of your waking hours spent in pursuit of a paycheck. I know that many of you work 60-h work weeks (or more) and that then has you providing care for over 53.5% of your waking hours. In many cases, we would gladly accept the opportunity to work fewer hours but current staffing shortages demand that we are more available to employers than what might be considered ideal. Even at 35% of our waking hours, our job occupies more time than what we are likely committing to our relationships, our families, our religion, our community service, or those activities that bring about a sense of well-being or happiness. So then, how much money is required to make this temporal sacrifice acceptable?

Perspective has a lot to do with what might be viewed as a reasonable salary, and compared to most people working outside of healthcare fields, healthcare professionals are generally compensated at a high level. In 2022–2023, inflation is running rampant so any discussion of salary will likely become moot in short order. However, in 2021 the median US salary for men was $50,391 and the median women's salary was $36,726 (Fool.com 2022). Not all healthcare workers can expect to greatly exceed these median salary numbers and, in some cases, may even fall short. Take nursing assistants, for example. In many cases, these professionals represent the institutional backbone that allows patients to have their basic needs met. The backbreaking work done by this group includes significant lifting, attendance to patient's personal needs, and may be incredibly physically demanding. Despite the critical value provided by this group, average reimbursement in 2022 sits at $33,250 (Joblist.com 2022). At this number, they are receiving a solid 10% less than the median US annual salary for women and significantly less than what I have seen posted for jobs at local franchised eating establishments. Nurses generally do significantly better with average salaries ranging from $72,260 to $85,020 depending upon a number of factors including geography and location of care provided (inpatient work is generally reimbursed at a higher rate than outpatient) (Joblist.com 2022). Finally, physicians encounter a huge range in reimbursement with average salaries for primary care doctors at $223,000 (Joblist.com 2022). There is then a large range within medical specialities. In each case, it is difficult to know exactly how worth and salary was historically determined but the upper range can be fairly astronomical. In 2022, 9 physicians were listed on the Forbes' list of billionaires with most of the tremendously high-level income being derived from industry or organizational leadership (Beckersasc.com 2022). While some practicing physician salary numbers may seem high, they generally pale in comparison to those no longer practicing medicine but occupying space in the ivory towers of our healthcare institutions. Healthcare CEO's can command significant salaries with one receiving more than $18 million dollars in 2018 alone (Healthaffairs.com 2022). Whatever the case and however these numbers came to rest where they have, we are all mortgaging some aspect of our lives to earn a living. Why present these numbers? Won't they only seek to create divisions between different groups of healthcare professionals? I really hope that this is not the case and, if anything, perhaps it serves to demonstrate/remind some of the higher wage earners that their work is only made possible by those earning a much smaller paycheck and that they might consider utilizing their influence to seek additional reimbursement opportunities for those at the lower end of the wage spectrum.

Our upbringing introduces an entirely different but equally powerful notion of what represents a reasonable annual salary. In early 2022, a Wharton professor queried her students on what they thought the average American earned over the course of a given year. Here is where perspective makes a huge difference – 25% of the students responded that they thought the average salary was greater than $100,000 per year. One seemingly privileged student responded that their approximation of the average US annual salary was $800,000 per year. The perspective of these students attending a prestigious (and expensive – the Wharton MBA program tuition and fees are listed as >$82,000 per year) business school demonstrates that it can be difficult to understand the perspective of others if their financial history and experience do not match your own. Wharton students are generally from families that are in the top 20% of earners (the average family income of a Penn student is $195,000) and therefore, it should not come as any great surprise that their students have limited insight into the financial situation of many of their peers (Phillyvoice.com 2022). Your personal experience with money might similarly be expected to impact your financial success and your satisfaction with the equation that leverages time for reimbursement. If you were raised in a family in the upper half of income generation, a recent Pew research study demonstrated that over half of your income generating potential is derived by factors that can be traced exclusively back to familial income (Pewtrusts.org 2022). However, there may be a hidden dark side to formative years spent living on financial easy street. A healthcare professional earning $200,000 per year in reimbursement may feel grossly undervalued when compared to the time and effort required to earn that salary if their parent's income exceeded one-million dollars per year. In the same vein, if your parents struggled with finances, you may find that the $200,000 annual salary has a very different appearance.

Oftentimes, the scale of a healthcare professional's debt, their income, and how best to navigate their finances can become overwhelming. For some, their lives have been dedicated to learning medicine and honing their skills caring for patients. Many healthcare professionals find that these skills are not enough and that they are ushered into their careers unprepared to simultaneously serve as small business owners. One thing that will not improve the financial outlook for any provider is to stick their head in the sand and hope that things will work out. There is power in education and we are now fortunate to live in an era where there are ample opportunities to obtain advice on financial matters. Unfortunately, our institutions of higher learning are generally doing a poor job preparing healthcare workers for their financial futures. In one study of over 2000 residents and fellows, 52% had not yet initiated retirement savings and 48% owed greater than $200,000 in education loans. Nearly 1/3 of participants in this study reported difficulty covering basic monthly expenses, 20% responded that they would carry a credit card burden at the end of the month, and those trainees with significant debt were generally less satisfied than those who were debt free (Ahmad et al. 2017). The power of education and the impact that financial education can have on healthcare professional well-being was demonstrated in a recent study that evaluated the impact of financial literacy courses provided to Obstetrician/Gynecologist residents and fellows. This study demonstrated that inclusion of these trainees in a five-part financial literacy course significantly improved their sense of well-being, their belief that they would meet their financial goals in a reasonable time, their working understanding of personal financial planning topics, and their understanding of the financial services industry (Cawyer et al. 2022). The power of financial education and literacy seems to garner significant attention among physicians but published literature remains much more muted in its advice to other medical professionals. This is unfortunate because what published literature does exist suggests that large numbers of our nursing colleagues feel uncertain in their finances and unprepared for retirement (Valencia and Raingruber 2010; Kowalski et al. 2006). A study of veterinary students found that those students with higher debt burden had decreased financial satisfaction and that decreased financial satisfaction was significantly correlated with depressive symptoms (Britt-Lutter and Heckman 2020).

The solidly good news is that there are abundant resources available to help and the vast proliferation of these resources likely means that there is some media that speaks to your exact situation. The abundance of podcasts that focus on finance topics is astounding and these resources allow for the passive absorption of information during your commute or morning run. With so many options to choose from, it may be difficult to know where to start your audio journey but pick one, give it a whirl, and if it doesn't resonate with you pick another. It seems that there are often recurrent themes on these podcasts or teachable moments that are important to the hosts. Therefore, changing your listening habits every so often may offer a fresh take on how to manage your finances that proves helpful. Beyond podcasts, there are blogs and internet postings from many of the same individuals. There have also been some fantastically well written books published recently that detail pathways to financial wellness. Finally, there are paid professionals who may be able to assist you in your financial wellness journey.

With many investment options (real estate, stocks, cryptocurrency, NFT's, etc.), finance management has the potential to become incredibly complicated. However, it seems that it does not need to be. Boiling down the financial advice doled out in various advice platforms usually leads to only a small number of similar overarching themes. First, these outlets generally recommend the elimination of debt. This certainly applies very strongly to high-interest credit card and education debt as they have the greatest potential to weigh down the accumulation of wealth. Beyond fiscal responsibility, the elimination of these debts can be emotionally satisfying. A recent survey of over 1000 student loan borrowers found that 61% feared that their student loan debt worries were spiraling out of control, 64.5% were losing sleep due to debt, and 67% were experiencing physical symptoms of anxiety related to this debt (headaches, muscle tension, upset stomach, rapid heartbeat, tremors, fatigue, and shortness of breath) (Lendingtree.com 2022). Prioritizing the payment of these loans and actively seeking out available forgiveness programs may have an outsized impact on the overall wellness of an individual beyond just their net worth. When high-interest debt has been managed, most experts seem to agree that creating an emergency reserve is a sound strategy to avoid once-again falling into the trap of high-interest loans. Another common piece of financial advice frequently retold is to maximize investments in tax-advantaged accounts and then focus on investments in risk-mitigating index funds. With these funds, an individual seems less likely to hit it rich but more likely to realize steady growth and avoid placing all their investment hopes in an individual company that may not be there in the future. Finally, when training is complete and you finally have that grown-up salary, work to avoid the lifestyle creep or steady increase in expenditures that have the potential to stymie your financial wellness progress. Try to remember how happy cheap pizza and a movie at home on a Friday night made you for the first 30 years of your life. Just because you now have that big paycheck, doesn't mean that you now need box theater seats. The hedonic treadmill is a theory that basically states that people have a baseline and steady level of happiness that they are destined to return to. Some of the purchases that we make may result in temporary augmentations of our happiness level but these are likely fleeting and the luster will be off of that new car long after it has ceased providing us with additional happiness. Finally, attempt to be content with what you have and avoid making material or experiential comparisons to others. The social comparison theory posits that we all gauge our personal and social worth based on how we stack up to others. At one point, we lived in smaller communities and it was easier to be the best at some activity or to have had some experience that set you apart. With the rampant use of social media platforms, it is far too easy to envy another individual who has taken better vacations than you, has a nicer house than you, or has accomplished something that shadows your own experiences. If possible, catch yourself if you see these comparisons diminishing your own happiness or driving you to seek ever more impressive (and expensive) pathways to social media distinction.

And with that, please keep in mind that *"The editor of this book is a practicing physician, author, and backyard farmer. They are not a licensed accountant, attorney, or financial advisor. So, this book is for your entertainment and information only and should not be considered official personalized financial advice."*

References

Ahmad FA, White AJ, Hiller KM, et al. An assessment of residents' and fellows' personal finance literacy: an unmet medical education need. Int J Med Educ. 2017;8:192–204.

Beckersasc.com. www.beckersasc.com/asc-news/9-physician-billionaires-on-forbes-2022-list.html. Accessed 25 Nov 2022.

Britt-Lutter S, Heckman SJ. The financial life of aspiring veterinarians. J Vet Med Educ. 2020;47(1):117–24.

Cawyer CR, Blanchard C, Kim KH. Financial literacy and physician wellness: can a financial curriculum improve an obstetrician/gynecologist resident and fellow's Well-being? AJP Rep. 2022;12:e64–8.

Edsurge.com. www.edsurge.com/news/2017-07-20-how-many-times-will-people-change-jobs-the-myth-of-the-endlessly-job-hopping-millennial. Accessed 25 Nov 2022.

Fool.com. www.fool.com/the-ascent/research/average-us-income. Accessed 25 Nov 2022.

Healthaffairs.com. http://www.healthaffairs.org/do/10.1377/forefront.20220208.925255/#:~:text= A%202021%20report%20from%20the,were%20paid%20on%20average%20 %24600%2C000. Accessed 25 Nov 2022.

Joblist.com. www.joblist.com/guides/average-healthcare-salaries. Accessed 25 Nov 2022.

Kowalski SD, Dalley K, Weigand T. When will faculty retire?: factors influencing retirement decisions of nurse educators. J Nurs Educ. 2006;45:349–55.

Lendingtree.com. www.studentloanhero.com/featured/psychological-effects-of-debt-survey-results. Accessed 25 Nov 2022.

Pewtrusts.org. www.pewtrusts.org/en/about/news-room/press-releases-and-statements/2015/07/23/
    parental-income-has-outsized-influence-on-childrens-economic-future. Accessed 25 Nov 2022.
Phillyvoice.com.   www.phillyvoice.com/penn-wharton-professor-nina-strohminger-viral-tweet-
    average-american-salary. Accessed 25 Nov 2022.
Valencia D, Raingruber B. Registered nurses' views about work and retirement. Clin Nurs Res.
    2010;19(3):266–88.
Whitecoatinvestor.com. www.whitecoatinvestor.com/opportunity-cost-roi-fellowships. Accessed
    25 Nov 2022.

Eureka!

14

Errin Weisman

After an exhausting day working at my outpatient family medicine clinic, I was once again the last parent to pick up my two boys from day-care. My husband was working late, so I was on my own. We drove home and I fed and bathed my little ones entirely on autopilot. They splashed around like Shamu in their bubble bath, giggling as I slumped by the side of the tub, waiting for the day to be over. Massaging the ever-present dull headache at my temples, I remember thinking, *"This is not what my motherhood was supposed to be like."*

Being a mom held a very special place on my checklist of a 'successful' life. From the moment I decided to go to medical school, I had it all planned out.

Diploma: Check
A supportive spouse who loves me as I am: Check.

Kids: Check
Big girl doctoring job that would save the world? On the surface, this looked like the final checkmark, but it didn't turn out quite how I expected.

The professional track that I had worked so long and hard for had turned from a dream to what felt like a nightmare. I had become a robot, working day in and day out, while my dream of helping others and making a big impact slowly eroded. That feeling followed me home. It didn't matter how loving my kids and husband tried to be, because I never had enough energy to be fully present. And yet, I kept holding onto this version of my life because it was what I had planned. I wanted to keep believing this was my calling, even though deep down, it wasn't serving me or my family.

Becoming a doctor was supposed to be the pinnacle of all my hard work in school and residency. It was supposed to bring me fulfilment and all the good 'feels.'

E. Weisman (✉)
Otwell, IN, USA
e-mail: hello@burntouttobadass.com

But I was running on fumes. I'd drop the kids off at day-care, commute to work still exhausted from the day before, down several cups of coffee, walk or jog during lunch (if I even got lunch), and then do the reverse 10–12 h later. Rinse and repeat daily.

The underlying truth here: *Life changed, but my plans didn't.*

I had mastered the art of ignoring the signs and was slowly going numb to everything except for the strongest of emotions. Sunday night was the worst of it and came with feelings of dread and despair. I was frustrated with how the healthcare system tried to fold me into knots instead of just doing and paying for what was right for my patients. I was frustrated by my day-to-day office flow and the disregard I faced as a physician because I was the junior in the group. I felt completely unseen and misused.

I was not able to be an employed full-time PCP who didn't ask questions. It's just not in my DNA. But, in my mind, this was a sacrifice I had to make for my family. There was a lot holding me back from being honest with myself, not least of which was that sweet, sweet physician's paycheck and the massive debt it was paying. These were my golden handcuffs. On top of that, the guilt. We had organized our lives so I could be a fully committed physician. My husband took the more "supportive parenting" role to be more available for our children. *How dare I change my career?*

We had both made huge compromises and sacrifices to get to where we were. We had a mountain of educational loans and little mouths to feed. It was the path I had chosen. *How dare I change my mind?*

Having children changed everything for me without me really knowing. They forced me to see that the path I was on was unsustainable. And it was my children, especially my oldest son, who were my inspiration and motivation to get my ass out of the rut and pursue a job that felt right for me. I wanted them to grow up and remember, *"Mom really liked what she did."*

I remember the evening well when my partner and I were sitting around our kitchen bar, after another torturous day, when I turned to him, voice shaking, and said, *"I'm quitting my job."* He took it well, all things considered. After all, he wanted me to be happy, and he could see the toll it was taking on me. So, he reassured me that we would figure something out. At first, I thought I would have to quit clinical medicine altogether. I wasn't alone there: a quick Google will tell you that nearly 40% of female physicians go part-time or quit within 6 years of completing their residency. There's a reason why mothers in medicine are burning out at almost twice the rate of males and non-parents and reporting high levels of workplace discrimination related to pregnancy and motherhood. This wasn't just a 'me' problem—it's systemic.

I started brainstorming alternatives. Pharm? Leaving medicine and trying a different industry? Work the checkout line at the local store, Rural King? All possible and yet it felt like I was running away more than running towards my next professional step. Working with a coach, I started off with a simple question: *What did I really enjoy doing?* Hm. I honestly couldn't think of more than 5 things. I had been so focused on career goals and fulfilling my medical destiny that I hadn't left time for much else, and there was no space for *enjoying* things. I just did what had to be done, whatever the cost.

So, I moved to write a different list, which I entitled, 'What I'll NEVER do again (unless we are homeless, eating cat food and desperate for cash)!' Well, for one thing, I decided that I never wanted to work on an RVU-based pay system again. That led to other Nevers: I would never give over my autonomy and control of my office schedule and call calendar. I would never put myself in a place where I was minimized for being young, a woman, pregnant, or inexperienced. I would never work for an organization that didn't value my opinion, listen to my concerns, support me as a mother, or refuse to make appropriate changes. I would never allow patients to treat me or my staff as less than. I realized my 'Never Again' list didn't include anything I did as a physician. It was all the other stuff. The bureaucracy and the 'earning your stripes' mentality that came with working in medicine. I loved talking with patients and colleagues. I loved being able to help guide patients on their health journey. I loved working with my hands-on procedures and OMT (osteopathic manipulation techniques). I loved working with a team, and I valued being able to help people with my knowledge.

That was my eureka moment. *I didn't have to leave medicine to be happy!*

What I did realize was that I needed to leave my practice, the full-time job I was doing. So that's what I did. Not immediately, but with small steps and a plan. I took the things I was good at in medicine (listening to patients, having difficult conversations, empathizing) and I realized I could embrace those qualities in a new direction: coaching. I could coach myself out of this horrible place, and I could use my experience and my expertise to help others do the same. Because throughout this whole thing, I had never felt more alone, and I never wanted anyone who was going through the same thing to feel as alone as I did.

It was a slow process, entering the entrepreneur space, building an online business from scratch while having little to no internet in rural Indiana. There were certainly times I thought it wasn't going to be okay. It's scary to strike out on your own, to forge a new path that looks nothing like the one you planned when you were eighteen. Especially when you're a Type-A, neurotic perfectionist.

But guess what? We were totally fine as a family. We worked it out. And I guess even if we hadn't, it would have been okay. In the wise words of Mr. Weisman, *"There's a doctor shortage. If things get bad, I bet you could always go back."* Even with that fallback, making such a big career move was nerve-wracking. No one teaches you how to adapt, even though we have to keep doing it time and time again. When I finally embraced this challenge to change, my life did a complete 180. And, boy, am I glad it did.

I learned that when you make big changes, you're not only making them for you. By taking care of yourself and making money in a way that brings you energy, joy and control, you're giving your kids a truly happy mom. Now, instead of rushing my kids to bed at night and out of bed in the morning, I cuddle with them every chance I get. Instead of blowing up at little inconveniences, I honor my capacity to practice patience, understanding, and forgiveness. I'm far from being a perfect mom. But making changes in my career allowed me to experience the joy of mothering. By letting go of the idea of motherhood that I had so desperately clung to, *I've become the mom that I wanted to be.*

More importantly, *I've become the person I wanted to be.* And my kids see that.

No paycheck is worth as much as having my son look me in the eyes and say what he said to me the other day. *"I'm glad that you're a happy mommy now."*

I had to go through…

Cranky Mommy.

Angry Mommy.

Numb Mommy.

Too-Flippin-Tired-Please-Don't-Talk-to-Me-Right-Now Mommy.

And

Very, Very Alone Mommy.

Sometimes these mommies show up again, but now, it's in small doses. Overall, I am truly a Happy Mommy now. And I've even returned to clinical practice, but now it's on my terms—working reasonable hours for me and my needs (which for me is about three and half days a week). I don't take unfinished notes home, skip lunch, or fixate on fixing everything every day. I do good work in the midst of chaos. I help my patients and staff even if it's just 10%. I use all my vacation days to recover and refresh. And therefore, every day I arrive at the practice feeling fresh, engaged, and able to support my patients. Don't get me wrong, there are still dumpster fires that happen on a regular basis. But the difference this time around is I know that this is what happens when life is wrong. It's not because I'm at fault, didn't plan enough or am lacking.

This is what life looks like when it's working.

You have done hard things in the past. You will continue to be able to handle hard.

Just keep going.

So, if you've been on the cusp of something similar, I encourage you to make that change. Take a break from what is causing you to feel wretched and towards what will help make your soul happier. You don't have to know the whole plan, just the first step.

Your family will thank you later.

Errin Weisman, DO (she/they/doctor) openly speaks on her experience of professional burnout early in herfamily medicine career so that no person feels alone and to prove you can have a joy-filled and sustainable career. Dr. Weisman is also a champion of people in rural Southwest Indiana in her clinical practice.

She is a mother of dragons, keeper of the Amazon account, and lover of all things animals and alpacas.

Besides being sassy, she enjoys getting mud on her boots, teaching her children to forage in the woods and reading a great fantasy fiction novel.

Enough

15

Chirag P. Shah and Jayanth Sridhar

Enough. Understanding the concept of enough and living by its tenets can allow one to achieve financial peace. Enough is a multifaceted philosophy. It means as much as needed … period. One needs enough food to thrive and survive; too little he starves, too much he feels bloated and fat. Likewise, we need enough money to live a good life. We need enough for the basics for sustenance, but we also need a little more to feel financially secure. The absolute value of enough varies per person. Some "need" to fly business class or buy a second home, while others are content with more humble needs.

It is critical to remember that enough is absolute, and not relative. It is so tempting to compare yourself to others who may make more or have more than you. This comparison can influence your definition of enough for yourself. Do not fall into this trap. Your enough is absolute, not relative to the next person. Once you make enough, or have enough, the rest is gravy. You can certainly spend or do more if you have extra discretionary resources, but your happiness and sense of contentment should be fulfilled with your absolute level of enough, while any excess is a bonus. If you are constantly trying to make or have more, constantly chasing a moving target, it is impossible to enjoy the peace inherent to having enough. Peace is a mindset, and a choice.

As healthcare professionals, we invest a whole lot of time and energy to practice our trade. Most of us incur significant financial debt and stress laboring through school in the hopes of matching into our desired residency or job. There is no such thing as a time debt, as the time we spend training is spent and does not return later; time is a nonfungible asset that we choose to invest into our professions. Ultimately, most doctors are rewarded both by the satisfaction of helping others and with a

C. P. Shah (✉)
Ophthalmic Consultants of Boston, Boston, MA, USA
e-mail: cshah@post.harvard.edu

J. Sridhar
Bascom Palmer Eye Institute, University of Miami, Miami, FL, USA

decent salary. But, perhaps shockingly, most doctors are not rich. Doctors make an average of $300,000 per year but the majority have a net worth less than $1,000,000. How could this be? There are likely numerous factors that contribute to our modest net worth. Doctors start their attending jobs later in life due to the years of medical school and training, and they do so with an average of $200,000 in debt. Further, we are ingrained with the concept of delayed gratification throughout medical school and residency, perhaps leading to explosive spending when we start earning an attending's salary. Societal expectations may also play a role in influencing doctors to live a doctor's life. Further, docs get little formal education in financial planning during their training.

You are familiar with the FIRE movement, or Financially Independent Retire Early. It is sad testimony about the field of medicine if one spends all that effort, time and money slogging through medical school and residency only to retire prematurely. Enjoy the ride, it only gets better. Perhaps a better movement is FINS, Financially Independent No Stress. We encourage you to achieve financial independence early in your career so that you may practice medicine on your own terms, without the stress of working for a paycheck. This will mean different things for different people. It might mean spending more time with less profitable endeavors, like mission work, teaching, or research. For us, it meant writing a book entitled *Financial Freedom Rx*, and teaching young doctors the formula to financial security. Or it could mean working fewer hours or fewer days, spending more time with family, friends, and your golf caddy. They say couples fight about many things, but it typically falls within three categories: family, intimacy, and money. With financial security, you can focus on the first two.

There are many financial uncertainties in life and in medicine. The COVID-19 pandemic impacted many fields of medicine, causing reduced patient volumes and revenue. Reimbursements tend to drop over time, and do not necessarily grow commensurate to inflation. Private equity acquisitions have infiltrated some fields, cutting future earnings in as much as half or more for young doctors. Mental and physical health can impact a physician's productivity. For these reasons, and undoubtedly more to come in the future, it is important to plant a money tree soon after medical school.

What is financial independence? It is freedom from a paycheck and from the financial stresses inherent to life. It is traditionally defined as accumulating 25 times one's annual expenses, which allows a 4% draw for 30 years. The sooner in life one achieves financial independence, the greater she must accumulate or the less she must draw.

How does a healthcare professional achieve financial independence? The traditional business model for healthcare professionals is to trade time for money. Work more, see more patients, do more procedures. All of this leads to a bigger paycheck. But this model is not sustainable. We get older. Reimbursements can drop. Overhead can rise. And before you know it you are running to stand still. We each need to plant a money tree that grows and bears fruit as we approach the middle and end of our working years. For most of us, this requires developing and nurturing a diversified investment portfolio.

With the same discipline that got you through school, you can achieve financial independence as a healthcare professional. The formula is not complex, just like losing weight = calories in calories out. Financial independence starts with budgeting so you understand your income and expenses. Then, determine how large you want to live and adjust your saving (and spending) rate appropriately. If you start your job with $250,000 of debt and save 20% of your gross earnings at a 4% real (inflation adjusted) rate of return, you will hit financial independence in 33 years. A 30% savings rate drops the interval to 21 years.

Of course, one's savings rate is inversely correlated with one's spending rate. If you save 20% ($60 K) of a $300 K paycheck and pay $40% in taxes ($120 K), you can spend the remaining 40% ($120 K) with impunity. But if you save 30% ($90 K) on a quest towards earlier financial independence and a more modest lifestyle, and pay the same amount in taxes, you are left with 30% ($90 K) to spend. This shrinks your lifestyle by 25%, or $30 K ($120 K - $90 K). That is a lot. But it comes back to the concept of enough. If you value the security of financial peace at a younger age, then you might also brown bag your lunch, metaphorically speaking, and live a happy life on a lower budget. But even if you "only" save 20% of your gross, you can sleep well knowing you are on track to achieving financial independence, likely around a traditional retirement age, while maximizing your lifestyle throughout your working years.

Healthcare professionals have the privilege of helping other people, often on patients' darkest days. As satisfying as this can be, it can also be draining after years of hard work and sacrifice. Healthcare professionals must care for themselves, physically, emotionally, mentally, spiritually, and financially, if they wish to care for patients. Our careers, though born through the sprints of medical/nursing/pharmacy/ dentistry/veterinary school and residency, take the form of a marathon when we ultimately finish our training. To succeed, we must pace ourselves, keep our chin up, and lungs full. Even just a small amount of financial planning—saving and investing 20%—allows one to live well on the remainder while having the peace of mind afforded by financial security. To achieve the happiness and contentment incumbent to enough, we must define enough for ourselves in absolute terms and enjoy the ride.

Financial Freedom Blueprint

16

Jordan D. Frey

Financial well-being is one of the most critical and often overlooked aspects of overall well-being for healthcare professionals. I personally experienced this at the end of my 7-year training period as a reconstructive plastic surgeon. I found myself burned out and losing my passion for medicine. Deep reflection helped me to identify that my lack of financial well-being was playing a huge role in my feelings of burnout. As a result, my wife and I made an effort to improve our financial well-being. As I continue on this path towards financial freedom, I have seen my overall well-being improve drastically. Equally as important is that I have re-discovered my passion for medicine and become a better physician in the process. This is something that we all can achieve.

Until I began caring for my financial well-being, personal finance intimidated and scared me. I had >$500,000 in student debt, credit card debt, no savings or investments, and no financial education. Unfortunately, this is not uncommon for many healthcare professionals. As a result, I stuck my head into the sand and ignored my finances. I fell victim to the all-too-common taboo in medicine that "money doesn't matter." While it is true that we get into this field to help others, as I have discovered, money does matter. It matters because our financial well-being affects our ability to care for patients. And financial freedom makes us better providers. In fact, imagine a country where every healthcare professional is financially free—working because he or she wants to, not because they have to. This would change our healthcare landscape for the better in ways that we cannot even yet imagine!

J. D. Frey (✉)
The Prudent Plastic Surgeon, Buffalo, NY, USA
e-mail: jordan@prudentplasticsurgeon.com

Regardless, your reason for improving your financial and overall well-being is personal. And perhaps you would like to reach financial freedom to leave medicine. There is nothing wrong with that. However, I imagine many of you, despite feelings of burnout, moral injury, fatigue, and loss of autonomy, would love to rediscover your passion for medicine on your own terms. This is exactly what financial freedom affords.

While I hope we have now established *why* financial well-being is important for healthcare professionals, it is important to address the *how*. As I mentioned above, personal finance and investing can seem complex, risky, intimidating, and scary. That is because we receive no formal financial education in our years and years of education and training. This is also to the benefit of salespeople often masquerading as financial "advisors," looking to take advantage of healthcare professionals.

The reality, however, is that personal finance is straightforward and simple. In fact, the fear I felt prior to looking at all of my financial mistakes soon turned to empowerment once I realized that I could now start to make positive changes. Your training in healthcare is much more challenging. If you can get through that, you can learn how to reach financial freedom!

Before diving deeper into the *how*, there is one other common limiting belief that I would like to address. All healthcare professionals, regardless of position or income, can achieve financial freedom. As I will show, your income level is just one of many variables in this equation. It is not the sole determinant. A family medicine doctor has the same ability as a plastic surgeon. A nurse has the same potential for financial independence as a physician. By following the simple personal finance principles herein, financial freedom is within your grasp!

12 Steps to Financial Freedom for Healthcare Professionals

Build Your "Why"

This is the most important step. It is the reason you want to achieve financial freedom and financial wellness. If there is no reason, then it will feel pointless when, and if, you get there. Any roadblock in the way will feel insurmountable. Your "why" is there to pull you through the hard times when you need it.

My "why" is that I want to gain financial well-being to enhance my overall well-being, to spend more time with my family and friends, and to pursue my passion on my own terms.

Begin Your Financial Education

Pick up a finance book. Start reading 10 pages each day, then try to read one financial book each year. It is minimal effort and will pay huge dividends in the long run. If you are not a fan of reading or want to get up to financial speed faster, I recommend podcasts or blogs.

Pay off Debt

This truly is the first step to financial freedom. You need to stop taking on new debt and get rid of any and all debt you currently have. When you are in a hole, the first step is to stop digging; then start climbing out. You can't run until you get out of the hole. Each $1 you use to pay off debt is another $1 increase toward achieving a positive net worth.

Get Insurance

If you depend on your income to live (i.e., you are not financially independent), then you need disability insurance. Does someone (i.e., spouse, kids) depend on your income to live? If so, you need term life insurance (not whole life insurance). Additionally, if you are practicing medicine, then you need malpractice insurance.

Not having sufficient coverage in these areas could set you and your loved ones up for potential financial catastrophe. Consider the idea that it is better to have it and not need it, than to need it and not have it.

Optimize Your Contract (Current or New)

Fair or not, contract negotiation is the time when you set the foundation for what you will make and how you will make it. There is usually some wiggle room within the contract to make more or less over time. However, you largely set the scale of your income as soon as you sign on the dotted line. Therefore, if you are negotiating your first contract, take the time to make it as favorable as possible. If you already have a contract, go through it and see what you would change if you could. See how close you are to your renewal time and create a strategy to make the next contract the best it can be.

Learn to Keep Score

One of the biggest mistakes that high income earners like healthcare professionals make is that we confuse income with net worth. And a high income does not guarantee a high net worth, i.e., wealth. If one makes $300,000 each year and spends $300,000 each year, their net worth and wealth is actually $0.

Net worth is calculated as the difference between your assets and your liabilities. Put simply, assets are things that put money in your pocket like stocks, bonds, and cash-flowing real estate. Liabilities meanwhile are things that take money out of your pocket like credit card debt, student debt, car loans, and personal home mortgages. This is why each $1 of debt paid off equals a $1 increase in your net worth.

Review your net worth at least every 2–3 months. See what actions are helping your net worth and which are hurting it. Then you can adjust your strategy.

Budget

Budgeting can seem quite restrictive. But in reality, it is the opposite. A budget allows us to track our spending to ensure that we can reach our financial goals. And it is very easy to do using the following steps:

- Come up with a list of broad categories of expenses (i.e., rent/mortgage, groceries, entertainment, taxes, etc.)
- Go to your bank account(s)/credit card(s) and put every single expense from the past month (first of the month to first of the month) in an expense category
- Add up the total for each expense category
- Add up the grand total for the month and make sure it is less (or at worst equal to) your monthly income
- Do you have enough left over to save for your financial goals?
- If yes, great! If not, what can you adjust to make this happen?
- Aim for a savings rate of at least 20%
- Now, go through each category and decide how much you can spend while still reaching your goals

The end goal of your budget is that you want to create a savings rate of at least 20% of your gross income. This savings rate is your margin, or the difference between what you earn and what you spend. And a simple formula to build wealth is to increase and invest your margin. Your budget helps you do exactly this.

Use the Right Strategy to Invest your Money

Once you have created a savings rate of at least 20% of your gross income, you need to invest that money. If you don't invest it, you are losing money due to inflation. The question then becomes, what is the best way to invest your money?

First, an important definition. A stock is a part ownership in a company. You buy one share and you become an owner. Each share has a price tag when you buy it that changes based on various and, at times, arbitrary factors as they are traded in the stock market.

When you buy a company's stock, you are saying that you believe in that company's success. If you are right, like with Apple, you make a lot of money. If you are wrong, like Enron, you lose all of your money. Picking the right company, or horse, can be difficult even for the "experts." Research shows that even "experts" underperform the overall stock market 80% of the time when they try to actively invest by timing the markets and picking stocks or funds.

When you buy the whole stock market, you are saying that you believe in the overall ingenuity and innovation of humankind and the world economy. This is a much safer bet. Over the long term, the overall stock market has always gone up. And you should only be investing money that you do not need in the short term. In this way, the short-term volatility of the stock market does not matter to you. You are now investing and not speculating.

You can invest in the overall stock market or large sectors of it using index funds. An **index fund** is a collection of stocks strategically picked to mirror some index marker of the overall stock market.[11] For instance, the S&P 500 is an index with a collection of stocks thought to give a good sense of the overall market. (Is the market going up or down? etc.) An index fund will mirror the movement of the index that it is based on.

You can also invest in index funds of bonds and even real estate, called Real Estate Investment Trusts, through just about any investment brokerage.

If you save 20% of your gross income and invest wisely in index funds, as a high-income earner, you will be able to retire and reach financial freedom on your own terms.

Invest in the Right Places

Once you have decided how to invest your savings, the next decision is where to invest your savings. You can invest in a regular taxable investment account. Money in this account is taxed when contributed (via income tax) and taxed again when it is withdrawn (via capital gains taxes).

However, there are other investment accounts available that carry significant tax advantages. These include 401 k, 403b, and 457 accounts. These are typically available through your practice or employer and are accounts that are not taxed upon contribution and only taxed upon withdrawal (tax deferred). Another available tax deferred investment account is an Individual Retirement Account or IRA. These accounts are available to anyone earning an income. However, most or all high income wage earners will be above the income limit to contribute to this account with a tax benefit. However, high income earners can still contribute to a "backdoor" Roth IRA in which your money is taxed upfront but never taxed again including upon withdrawal.

The best strategy is to maximize contributions to tax-advantaged accounts available to you before utilizing a taxable investment account.

Spend Intentionally

Intentional spending is the concept that one is intentional with the money that she or he spends. Meaning that any purchase is well thought out and carries an intended purpose. In contrast, unintentional spending is a reflex when money is spent without focusing on the joy, or lack thereof, it brings. Unfortunately, research has shown that we are incredibly bad at predicting what will make us happy—especially with our purchases. Therefore, it is important to mindfully practice intentional spending.

Here is a simple formula:

If a purchase meets *both* of these criteria:

- The purchase fits into your financial plan and
- The joy derived from the purchase is $\geq$ the dollar value of the purchase

You should buy it.

If the purchase meets *either* of these criteria:

- The purchase does not fit into your financial plan and
- The joy derived from the purchase is $<$ the dollar value of the purchase

You should not buy it.

Money is simply a tool. A tool that I believe should be used for the betterment of yourself, your loved ones, and your world community. Spending money that you would not miss is not bad. But at the same time, to spend that money unintentionally in a way that does not accomplish those goals would be wasteful. So, the key is to spend money intentionally.

K.I.S.S

We all know people in healthcare that are complexifiers. And we know those that are simplifiers. In general, it is the simplifiers who are able to break down difficult concepts into understandable and teachable components. Finance is no different.

Seek financial mentors who are able to simplify the concepts of wealth building. If you can understand and practice as a healthcare professional, you can understand and enact health financial strategies. If someone is explaining an investment that you cannot understand, it is best to avoid it.

Create a Written Personal Financial Plan

A written personal financial plan is a document that you create to guide your financial decisions based on your personal goals. With a financial plan, you can constantly refer back when faced with tempting or challenging financial decisions to ensure that you make the right ones—which will be completely personal to you. Creating a written personal financial plan is the culmination of each of the previously discussed steps.

To begin making your personal financial plan, list out your financial goals. Some examples are:

- Pay off consumer debt in 2 years
- Pay off student debt in 5 years
- Achieve a net worth of $1 million in 12 years
- Save enough to cash flow at least $250,000 in retirement (goal retirement at least by the year 20XX)
  - This will be via a hybrid approach using equity and real estate investing
  - Save $1–two million in equities for 4% yearly withdrawal of ~$71,000
  - Cash flow >$200,000 from real estate investments in 5 years
- Save $400,000 for kids' college

Everyone's goals should be different and unique to your own philosophy and circumstances. Once you have established these goals, create financial priorities or steps that will serve as signposts on your journey. Some examples:

- Pay down high interest debt (>8%)
- Establish emergency fund (3–6 month's expenses)
- Maximize 401 k retirement account
- Contribute to 529 college savings account
- Maximize 457(b) retirement account
- Pay down medium interest loans (6–8%)
- Contribute to back door/spousal Roth IRA (every January if contributing—2 steps)
- Contribute to retirement taxable account
- Pay extra to mortgage
- Pay down low interest loans (<3%)
- Donate to charity with equity dividends

Now create guidelines for how you will invest to reach these goals. That way, you know exactly what you need to do. After this, all you need to do is follow the plan and you will reach financial freedom. Here are some example guidelines:

- Our primary equity investment vehicles will be stock index mutual funds and bond index mutual funds, preferably within tax-sheltered accounts
  - In general, we will favor passively managed investments over actively managed investments
  - Our asset allocation will be 75% stocks, 25% bonds
  - We will rebalance back to this allocation once a year
- In a market downturn or bear market, we will not panic and sell low; however, we will try to use any truly extra cash (not emergency fund, etc.) to rebalance by buying more stock (or other depressed equity)

With a written financial plan, you have laid out your goals as well as general and specific directions for getting there. That's the hard part. Now, all that you have to do is implement the plan in an emotionless and mindless fashion and you can rest assured that we will reach our goals.

Personal finance is an important but all too overlooked component of personal well-being for healthcare professionals. By enacting simple and reproducible strategies, like saving and investing, all healthcare professionals can improve their financial well-being, reach financial freedom, re-discover their passion for medicine, and work on their own terms.

Utilizing My Medical Degree in Biopharma

17

Nerissa C. Kreher

"Oh no…"

The first words out of the mouth of the Pediatric Endocrinology Section Head at Massachusetts General Hospital when I called to tell her my husband had matched in Sports Medicine at MGH and I would love to take the Clinical Research position that I had interviewed for months prior.

The position had been cut and was no longer available. They had another role to offer; not in clinical research, but instead as a clinician seeing patients 80% of the time (and "don't worry, you will still have time to do research").

Throughout my fellowship training, I learned that clinical research was my passion. I attempted a basic science research career, working in my mentor's basic science lab; that was not for me! I had the opportunity to complete my Master's in Clinical Research via a NIH T32 grant and through that program was engaged in a clinical research project of my own. I developed the protocol, recruited patients, conducted the study, analyzed and published the results. These were the patients I enjoyed seeing. My general endocrinology clinic time was often tedious and fatiguing but my clinical research visits were invigorating.

Thus, when MGH offered me a clinical role, I knew in my heart that it was not for me.

As a pediatric endocrinologist, I needed to be in a specialized children's hospital. There are two in the Boston area and the other hospital was not hiring pediatric endocrinologists. I looked as far away as Rhode Island and New Hampshire and did not find an option that offered clinical research.

At the same time, a sales representative for a pharmaceutical company who was an acquaintance asked me to have lunch. During that lunch I explained my situation and the quandary our young family found ourselves in given my need for a job to

N. C. Kreher (✉)
The Pharma Industry MD Coach, Reading, MA, USA
e-mail: nkreher@iupui.edu

support our family in this move to Boston. She asked me to share my resume with her and she would share it at the company where she worked to see if they had an opening for a physician with my expertise.

And, I was asked to interview (!!) for a Medical Director, Medical Affairs job, supporting the Endocrine Business Unit. My expertise in pediatric endocrinology, specifically growth disorders and their treatment, were aligned with the company's needs. I worked with a recruiter that helped to prepare me for interviews; explaining who I would be meeting with, what questions they would likely ask, and what they would be assessing for.

Ultimately, I received a job offer and agreed to move to Boston and start the job a couple of months prior to our family moving. I was hooked from day one. I enjoyed so many things about the new role. In this new role I learned about marketing and regulatory, used my medical expertise to completely revise and re-launch a patient registry, and interacted with international and national thought leaders in the area of growth disorders and growth hormone treatment.

The Medical Affairs role involves communicating a company's science and clinical data to external stakeholders such as physicians. In addition, obtaining information from thought leaders about the diseases and therapies a company is working on and incorporating this clinical feedback into all work being accomplished at a company is critical to advancing medicine. These "scientific communications" can be accomplished through activities such as advisory boards, conferences and symposia, and publications. Medical Affairs may also be engaged, as I was, in phase 4 clinical registries. I was charged with re-invigorating a growth hormone registry that was not being utilized to its full potential. I was also involved in the clinical development of a growth hormone delivery device. Every day allowed for a variety of learning opportunities and I was constantly exposed to new concepts. Travel was a major part of this job and did require me to balance this requirement with caring for two young children at home; I am grateful I was able to have a live-in au pair to help our young family make this major transition.

My lessons learned from this transition into the biopharma industry include the following:

1. **Always network!** My acceptance of a lunch invitation turned into a job offer. Keep an open mind and engage with people on a regular basis.
2. **Be honest with yourself about what you enjoy**. What fulfills you? What do you enjoy? What do you avoid? Using this knowledge and honesty with myself to recognize I wouldn't be happy in a clinical role was critical to my ultimate transition.
3. **Take a chance.** I truly had no idea what Medical Affairs was when I was asked to interview for this job. I did not have experience in the pharmaceutical industry. I could have talked myself out of even trying… not even taken the interviews. Let go of fear getting in the way of possibility.

I have now worked in the biopharma industry for 17 years and in that time my experience includes both Medical Affairs and Clinical Development roles and the combination of the two has led to the role of Chief Medical Officer. In each role I have gained more and more experience and exposure and advanced from Medical Director to Senior Medical Director to Executive Medical Director and then to Vice President.

The Clinical Development role involves all things related to conducting clinical research. Common responsibilities include protocol development, interacting with regulatory/health authorities and discussing clinical development plans with experts in the therapeutic area. All roles in biopharma typically require cross-functional work and clinical development is no different. We work with team members including toxicology, pharmacokinetics, regulatory, statistics, medical writing, patient advocacy and commercial.

Many people ask me if I miss seeing patients. I don't; but remember that I never planned to see patients as the primary focus of my career. I am still connected with patients and families. My entire career has been focused on rare disease drug development. In the rare disease world, we meet patients and families to understand their disorders and incorporate their input into our development planning. Although I am not providing clinical care, I am still connected. I also still use my medical degree every single day. Whether it is educating colleagues about a disease that might be the target for a novel therapeutic or considering the appropriate inclusion and exclusion criteria for a clinical trial, my medical training is essential.

Biopharma careers are something that any physician can consider. Although we do not learn much, if anything, about this career option during medical school and residency, the pharma industry needs physicians to help conduct drug development activities. There are important responsibilities from early in the development process, even before the drug has been studied in human subjects, to after a drug has been approved for use by regulatory authorities. I encourage physicians to consider the option of biopharma as they evaluate the career path they will pursue.

My lessons learned after working in biopharma for more than 17 years:

1. There are **three main roles** for physicians entering the biopharma industry: Clinical Development, Medical Affairs and Pharmacovigilance (also called Patient or Drug Safety)
2. Despite many job descriptions asking for some number of years of experience working in pharma, I encourage physicians to apply for jobs that ask for less than 5 years of experience in pharma. You have to start somewhere and your medical training is the most critical part of the experience needed in biopharma.
3. Recognize that working in pharma requires cross-functional team work. You must be flexible and willing to listen and learn from others on the team.

Working in the biopharma industry is a remarkable way to use your medical degree. You are helping to bring new therapies to patients. You are educating others about diseases. The opportunities to learn new things and be challenged abound.

Part IV

Spirituality

Abstract

Within the practice of medicine, there are a spectrum of parameters and outcomes that seem beyond our reason to understand. Why do some patients contract and succumb to various diseases/conditions while others seem to defy the odds and rally? Why do members of our community commit atrocious acts and why do the most vulnerable seem most likely to suffer? For many, there is incredible solace that can be found in the various forms of spirituality that may assist in ascribing meaning and design to outcomes beyond our reasoning or control. However, the reality is that healthcare professionals struggle with the notion of spirituality and there are well-documented divides between the relationship that the general public versus scientists have with God. Beyond a relationship with the divine, there are mindfulness and meditation practices that may serve as spiritual substitutes/adjuncts and these practices may offer many of the same benefits associated with a religious affiliation.

Keywords: Faith; Compassion; God; Mindfulness; Meditation

Thought Questions:

1. What is your personal history with spirituality? Reflect on positive and negative experiences and consider if greater involvement/engagement might be a net positive endeavor. If your previous history with spirituality was negative, do the same conditions currently exist or have they changed in some substantial manner that might allow for re-exploration?

2. Can you recall a profoundly negative patient outcome for which you place significant blame on yourself or after which you are unable to effectively move on? Would ascribing some responsibility outside of yourself allow for personal healing and a greater ability to care for patients in the future?

3. Recall a time when you were asked to engage in prayer with a patient or family. How did you respond to this request, how did the request make you feel, and are you satisfied with your response? If/when you were to again receive this prayer request, how would you now respond?

4. Were you to further engage within a spiritual community, what benefits do you think that you might be able to effectively realize? For example, are there opportunities to benefit from an enhanced social support network, stress mediation outlet, or further connections with the patients and families within your sphere of care?
5. Recognizing that, for a variety of entirely legitimate reasons, organized religion may not be for everyone, are there mechanisms through which you might achieve a higher level of mindfulness?
6. Reflecting upon the normal workflow of your day, are there opportunities to introduce some mindfulness or meditation practices that might be of benefit to you and your colleagues?

Spirituality in Healthcare

18

Michael J. Gyorfi

Healthcare professionals accompany their patients as they experience pain, distress, functional impairment, and doubt resulting from illness and injury. Acting as an effective healer requires empathy and acknowledgment of the patient's experience. This empathy can be internalized and have a negative impact on the healthcare professional which is often termed "compassion fatigue". A meta-narrative by Sinclair, et al looked at 90 studies comparing compassion fatigue in various healthcare professions. Their findings emphasized common findings of compassion fatigue over numerous healthcare professions that were unrelated to their level of direct "compassionate care" suggesting that all healthcare professionals are at risk (Sinclair et al. 2017). However, flagging compassion levels are not the only culprit in the epidemic of healthcare professional burnout and exodus from the profession. Therefore, conceiving pathways to enhance healthcare professional compassion reserves, enhance resiliency, and decrease burnout have emerged as compelling societal needs.

In 1995, the World Health Organization declared that a patients' spirituality should be further recognized as a significant component of their quality of life. Spirituality is a broad and complex concept which varies in meaning according to different cultural, religious, and academic backgrounds. Historically, the term spirituality was used to describe the practices of people who dedicated their lives into religious services or exemplify the teachings of their faith traditions (Koenig 2008). Only in the last decades has spirituality been detached from religiosity as a distinct construct, even though the scientific community still refers to this research field using the "dual" term religiosity/spirituality. Despite having numerous definitions, the common backbone is often related to a dynamic and intrinsic sense of connection to something larger than oneself.

M. J. Gyorfi (✉)
University of Wisconsin School of Medicine and Public Health, Madison, WI, USA
e-mail: mgyorfi@uwhealth.org

Published research has demonstrated that including spiritual care in nursing practice benefits patients and the nurses caring for them through increases in professional satisfaction (Vlasblom et al. 2011). A review of 18 articles focusing on burnout and spirituality in nurses revealed that nursing professionals frequently turn to spirituality or religion as a coping mechanism for stress and burnout. Fifteen of the studies demonstrated lower levels of burnout, exhaustion, and depersonalization in various contexts associated with increased spiritual and religious beliefs. However, two studies failed to find a connection, and one found worse results (De Diego-Cordero et al. 2022).

A 2013 study further evaluated the correlation between burnout and spirituality. In this study, 259 medical students completed a survey which included measures of spirituality, burnout, psychological distress, coping, and general happiness. They found a significant inverse correlation between spirituality and measures of psychological distress/burnout paired with a positive correlation between life satisfaction and spirituality (Wachholtz and Rogoff 2013). In other words, increased spirituality resulted in less psychological distress as well as improvements in life satisfaction. Another survey study of 173 internal medicine and medicine/pediatric residents produced similar results with a strong correlation between spirituality and personal accomplishment (Doolittle et al. 2013). These results suggest that having a strong spiritual foundation and regular spiritual experiences is related to having a higher quality of life, less psychological distress, and less burnout. Of significant importance, high levels of spirituality appear to guard against learner burnout in the medical field and may serve as a mechanism to protect this more vulnerable group.

A large systematic review identified 493 articles that addressed spirituality and the impact that it can have in a healthcare setting. This review cast a wide net and included published work on spirituality for health care providers, patients, and the interaction between the two. It concluded that spirituality provides a framework for both providers and their patients that can significantly impact resilience and satisfaction. The discussion in this manuscript highlighted their difficulties studying such a broad and poorly defined concept and how augmenting their findings with strong statistical differences was challenging (de Brito Sena et al. 2021). However, this extensive review supports a growing body of research on the positive effects of spirituality and highlights its applicability as a potential method of healthy coping for all health care professionals. The study has additional implications for how increased training efforts and innovative facilitation of various spiritual expressions (such as inclusive forms of ritual recognition of loss) in the workplace might reduce the stresses of such work.

A further inspection of the PubMed database reveals that a staggering 30,000 research articles were published between 1999 and 2012 on the subject of spirituality in medicine (Lucchetti and Lucchetti 2014). However, a closer inspection of the available literature reveals that spirituality in healthcare is most often studied as a component of patient wellness and one of the factors that might significantly impact healthcare outcomes. It can be a tremendous struggle to identify large bodies of research attempting to evaluate the impact of spirituality on the healthcare professional as it seems to be a topic that is far less frequently addressed.

So then, why do healthcare professionals seem less willing to research or commit to considering how a foundation and commitment to spirituality might impact their wellbeing? For whatever reason, there often seems to be a disconnect or barrier that limits the ability to foster this spiritual connection. It is possible that this connection has been beaten out of those who too steadfastly seek solutions and pathways that are conducive to evaluation and review. If it can't be tested or if there can't be some sort of high-level statistical analysis applied, then these components of wellness are frequently disregarded. A 2009 Pew Research Center trial revealed that only 33% of scientists believe in God versus 83% of the general public. A full 41% of scientists have no belief in a higher power versus 4% of the general public (Pewresearch.org 2022). This is a foundational approach and belief system with significantly deep roots that anecdotally trace back to the Napoleonic era. At that time, French scientist Pierre-Simon Laplace had recently completed a book describing the creation of the universe and was set before Napoleon to discuss the text's merits. Though historical reports vary, Napoleon asked Laplace why the creator (God) failed to gain mention in Laplace's text describing the origins of the universe. By some accounts, Laplace replied—*"Je n'avais pas besoin de cette hypothèse-là"* or *"I had no need of that hypothesis."* (Wikipedia.org 2022) More recent popular literature has also evaluated the scientific community's relationship with the divine. In Jurassic Park, Michael Crichton wrote - *"God creates dinosaurs, God kills dinosaurs, God creates man, man kills God, man brings back dinosaurs."* The scientific and healthcare professional community may benefit from considering why their belief in a power beyond themselves is so much less prevalent than the general communities and if this belief system is contributing to the rampant problems of burnout and career satisfaction seen in this group.

If the need for God has been supplanted in medicine, is there any meaning or reason for what healthcare professionals witness on a daily basis. In worst case scenarios, a healthcare professional might assume that their actions and insight are solely responsible for patient related outcomes. On the one hand, this approach might lead to grossly overinflated egos and sense of responsibility for positive patient outcomes. Consider this quote from the 1993 movie thriller Malice –

The question is, 'Do I have a 'God Complex'?…which makes me wonder if this lawyer has any idea as to the kind of grades one has to receive in college to be accepted at a top medical school. Or if you have the vaguest clue as to how talented someone has to be to lead a surgical team. I have an M.D. from Harvard, I am board certified in cardio-thoracic medicine and trauma surgery, I have been awarded citations from seven different medical boards in New England, and I am never, ever sick at sea. So, I ask you; when someone goes into that chapel and they fall on their knees and they pray to God that their wife doesn't miscarry or that their daughter doesn't bleed to death or that their mother doesn't suffer acute neural trauma from postoperative shock, who do you think they're praying to? Now, go ahead and read your Bible, Dennis, and you go to your church, and, with any luck, you might win the annual raffle. But if you're looking for God, he was in operating room number two on November 17, and he doesn't like to be second guessed. You ask me if I have a God complex? Let me tell you something: I am God.

Components of this dialogue are certainly present in current medical practice. No matter the specialty, we are all intellectually gifted and exceptional relative to our societal peers. No matter the specialty, getting to the point where one has completed medical training conveys a certain level of dedication and constitutional stoutness. And our patients generally appreciate these attributes in our colleagues above their commitment to any component of spirituality. It is tremendously common to be asked about the skill of a surgeon or nurse. What are their outcomes, how often do they miss on an IV-line insertion, or are they a skilled proceduralist? However, an incredibly uncommon question centers around the spirituality of the healthcare professional. Our patients have unknowingly reinforced the notion that healthcare professionals operate outside of the spiritual realm and that outcomes are now derived from the person and not the divine.

On the other hand, this approach fails to acknowledge or allow for outcomes that are beyond our reasoning or that may only occur out of an abundance of luck (or lack thereof). As usurping gods, healthcare workers are exposed to feelings of guilt, shame, inadequacy, etc and therefore any individual masquerading as God in the healthcare setting is exposing themselves to significant danger. It is far too easy to fall prey to becoming overly proud of our "technological terrors." In an era where machines and monitors seem able to diagnose and address nearly every malady that might be thrust upon our patients, it is important to remember that there is a time for everyone and that the fates will at some point trim the thread of life for all of our patients. As much as we are unable to eliminate all fatalities from lightning strikes, we need to accept a certain level of morbidity and mortality and release ourselves from the burden of all blame associated with these outcomes. Spirituality is an open-source resource that is available to everyone and in some cases may offer the ability to provide context and meaning to adverse events and a framework for accepting what cannot be changed. Because one pathway to spirituality did not perfectly fit with an individual does not mean that there is not a potential pathway to a divine connection. There is a whole world of spiritual options to consider that may prove to be a better match than what may not have worked in the past.

The thing is… spirituality can be incredibly difficult. Minds that have been crafted for asking questions and seeking truth may find religion to be a stifling quagmire that fails to provide a reasonable answer. Beyond that, it can be difficult to identify a divine reason for the terrible outcomes, the lives tragically cut short, and the capacity for humans to inflict harm on others. For those struggling with these barriers, mindfulness and meditation may offer some of what is lacking when spirituality is not tenable. The practice of mindfulness aims for an individual to become more fully present and aware of their emotions, thoughts, senses and what they are experiencing. Through these processes, practitioners of mindfulness are able to achieve self-acceptance while decreasing stress and burnout. While research on this subject is not yet incredibly robust, a growing body of publications supports the routine implementation of mindfulness practices for healthcare professionals.

References

de Brito Sena MA, Damiano RF, Lucchetti G, Peres MFP. Defining spirituality in healthcare: a systematic review and conceptual framework. Front Psychol. 2021;12:756080. https://doi.org/10.3389/fpsyg.2021.756080.

De Diego-Cordero R, Iglesias-Romo M, Badanta B, Lucchetti G, Vega-Escaño J. Burnout and spirituality among nurses: a scoping review. Explore (NY). 2022;18(5):6.

Doolittle BR, Windish DM, Seelig CB. Burnout, coping, and spirituality among internal medicine resident physicians. J Grad Med Educ. 2013;5(2):257–61. https://doi.org/10.4300/JGME-D-12-00136.1.

Koenig HG. Concerns about measuring "spirituality" in research. J Nerv Ment Dis. 2008;196(5):349–55. https://doi.org/10.1097/NMD.0b013e31816ff796.

Lucchetti G, Lucchetti ALG. Spirituality, religion, and health: over the last 15 years of field research (1999–2013). Int J Psychiatry Med. 2014;48:199–215.

Pewresearch.org. https://www.pewresearch.org/religion/2009/11/05/scientists-and-belief/. Accessed 31 Dec 2022.

Sinclair S, Raffin-Bouchal S, Venturato L, Mijovic-Kondejewski J, Smith-MacDonald L. Compassion fatigue: a meta-narrative review of the healthcare literature. Int J Nurs Stud. 2017;69:9–24. https://doi.org/10.1016/j.ijnurstu.2017.01.003. Epub 2017 Jan 12

Vlasblom JP, van der Steen JT, Knol DL, Jochemsen H. Effects of a spiritual care training for nurses. Nurse Educ Today. 2011;31(8):790–6. https://doi.org/10.1016/j.nedt.2010.11.010; Epub 2010 Dec 10.

Wachholtz A, Rogoff M. The relationship between spirituality and burnout among medical students. J Contemp Med Educ. 2013;1(2):83–91. https://doi.org/10.5455/jcme.20130104060612.

Wikipedia.org. https://en.wikipedia.org/wiki/Pierre-Simon_Laplace. Accessed 31 Dec 2022.

The Constancy of Faith

19

Tamara Chambers

During the journey of life, traveling through hard times is inevitable. Whether the challenge is encountered at home, work, or in your personal life, each circumstance changes who we are from that day onward. We can allow hardships to bring us down or we can use the lesson or experience to help us become the best version of ourselves. In a world of constant change, I realized the only constant is my faith in God. While facing hardships, I am comforted by His consistency, love, and most importantly His grace. No matter if we doubt, forget, or veer off the religious journey, He is always there, no matter what.

I want to preface this chapter by stating that my faith and Christian journey has not been perfect or constant. In fact, there were years when I lost touch with my faith. However, I was honored to write this chapter to share my personal experience on how religion has impacted my resilience and share how it has played a pivotal role in both my personal and professional life.

My faith grew tremendously during the journey of having kids. I can remember it like it was yesterday. The day I had been looking forward to for years, especially the last 9 months. There I was, laying on the labor and delivery bed as I just delivered my first child and waiting for the nurse to put my little girl on my chest for the very first time. However, instead of holding her within minutes of birth, she was quickly taken to the infant warmer and resuscitation efforts began. This was a distinct moment in time when I felt completely helpless. I could have screamed, cried, yelled, demanded things of the medical team, but instead I laid there quietly and prayed. I was extremely anxious about this pregnancy and delivery since I had already lost my first child to miscarriage. To ease my anxiety, I elected to listen to Christian worship music during my delivery to provide some calm and peace through the birthing process. As I laid there, watching them resuscitate my little girl, the song "God, I Need You" by Matt Maher played. It was at that moment, through

T. Chambers (✉)
Chief Clinical Officer, Grant Regional Health Center, Lancaster, WI, USA
e-mail: tchambers@grantregional.com

those words, that I had overwhelming peace overcome me as I was reminded that only He had control of this situation and I needed His help no matter the outcome of the situation.

This was only one of many difficult moments in my life when feelings of extreme exhaustion and being overwhelmed have caused me to lean on my faith and ask for help from God. My faith journey is not perfect. I do not go to church every Sunday, nor have I read the Bible from cover to cover, but I do know the truth that my faith is my foundation. My faith is the only source of constant consistency, comfort, and unending love and grace. My faith provides me with a never-ending source of comfort, love, and grace.

Faith has also taught me coping mechanisms and allowed me the opportunity to look at life through a different lens. When things are difficult, frustrating, or do not make sense, I challenge myself to consider the potential purpose behind these obstacles. At times, the answer is clear while at other times the answer appears many years later. Believing that everything happens for a reason and for a purpose provides comfort, peace, and hope.

The pandemic had a tremendous impact on my faith journey as well. One year before the pandemic hit, I transitioned into my first executive job in a new hospital. Knowing I was new at the position and had much more to learn, I found myself allowing fear and doubt to cloud my vision for my career. I felt unworthy and incapable of being successful or helping others. These feelings quickly lead to feelings of wanting to give up and walk away from the profession. I know I am not alone with that thought, as I have heard many health care professionals pondering that dangerous thought during the pandemic. We dedicate lots of money, time, and effort building our careers and it was depressing that I felt it was easier to just walk away. After an exhausting and extremely challenging day, when I constantly questioned if the actions taken that day were the right actions to protect and support the staff and patients, some small gesture would remind me of God's plan, grace, and love. For example, during one of the most horrible weeks of my career, one email from a nurse changed my outlook and caused me to refocus. Her message was simple yet impactful and the timing was absolutely perfect. Her message read: *"I just wanted you to know I see you ...... I see you taking each day in stride... I see you not knowing all the answers to the questions (because right now no one does know). But I see you smile and say we will try to find the answer. I see you and the admin team being, more than ever, on call to your staff on the front line. And even though you may not be the one donning the PPE and entering those rooms, you are still trying to protect your staff. Just wanted you to know I am thankful that you are in the position you are in - a position that may not be thanked enough."* This nurse granted me grace when I was not giving it to myself. Some may view the timing of this message as a coincidence, but to me and because of my faith, I saw it much differently. To me, her message was a reminder from Him and she was the messenger.

The ultimate grace giver is God. I read a quote from Joel Osteen recently that said *"His grace doesn't mean He's going to remove the challenge; it doesn't mean the opposition is going to let up. It means He's going to increase your strength so that it doesn't feel as difficult. As you get stronger, what you're up against becomes easier. God won't always lessen what's coming against you; He'll add to your strength."* This message is comforting to me during difficult times. It is unrealistic to believe the remainder of our career will be without challenge or hardship, but if you believe in God and accept His grace, you will come out stronger on the other side.

In addition to unfailing love, a relationship with God offers amazing grace. Experiencing His grace in my imperfect life, has changed me. Now, providing grace to others is one of my core values. Life is hard and we do not know the battles others face. However, we have the power to be kind and provide grace to others in all situations. When we are having a bad day or are struggling to resolve a conflict or challenge, would you rather someone tell you *"I see you. I know you don't have the answers and that is okay, you will in time"* or that *"you will never be good enough."* We all struggle, we all doubt. Why don't we overcome those feelings by being kind to one another and offering grace? Through grace, comes hope. And out of hope, comes love. Jesus was the ultimate granter of grace. His disciples sold him out prior to His death but He forgave them even before they betrayed Him. How powerful is that? What a phenomenal teacher He is for all of us. Grace is not only something to be granted to others as a show of kindness and support, but it is also needed for self-care.

So, whenever you feel dissatisfied with your professional impact or performance or the life you live outside of work, grant yourself some grace. You do not expect others to be perfect and have it together all the time, so stop expecting that of yourself. When faced with difficulty, remind yourself that the situation is tough, but so are you. You may not be able to control a situation, but you have the power to control how you respond. See challenges as lessons, seek to learn, improve each day, step by step, and rely on God for His help, support, and guidance.

My faith has also caused me to pause, be thankful, and take in the little moments especially after the pandemic hit. Moments found in the perfect stillness of a sunset can provide peace and hope for a better tomorrow, even if the day was unbearable. At the conclusion of every day, I have experienced benefits from entering in a journal three good things from each day. This practice instills gratitude and reflection into my daily routine. From a fun memory made with my kids, to a sincere thank you from a patient or staff member, it is powerful to reflect on the positive moments that might be too easily missed. If you take time to look, it is easy to identify those moments.

I feel blessed to have been called into the profession of healthcare to live out my mission to positively impact the lives of those I serve. However, I recognize I would not be successful without the foundation of my faith. You may not be where you want to be yet in life, but you are also not where you used to be. Take a second to realize how far you've come and grant yourself some grace, you deserve it.

Becoming Less Fantastic

20

Matt Norvell

To survive as a professional working in the healthcare context, I have decided to adopt a possible heresy: It is okay to be a little bit less fantastic.

I know that some people cannot make sense of that sentence. Some naturally and effortlessly ooooze fantasticness and wonderment and high achievement and cannot turn it off. But for the rest of us, it is easy to feel like we need to keep striving to be the "best of the best" all the time in every aspect of our lives. And the pressure of these expectations, both internal and external, is taking its toll.

Most of us came into healthcare to be fantastic, to be at the head of our class, and to push the various envelopes of innovation. Most of us also have the internal motivation to be generally good and healthy people who hope to be excellent parents or spouses or friends or siblings. I see you marathon runners and bike riders out there. I see you folks juggling three and five grants at a time. I see those of you who go to three grocery stores so you can have a perfectly nutritionally balanced meal for your family. We did not show up to be "good enough."

Here in late 2022, part of our current challenge is that we cannot do things exactly as we would normally want to do them. We know the right staffing ratios, we know the preferred parenting techniques, we know how we would be the ideal nurse or doctor or administrator or researcher or chaplain if the circumstances allowed. It is easy for any of us to get drawn into the idea that the only way to do something is at its highest, most excellent, exactly right, most fantastic level and anything short of that is failure. However, circumstances have changed and they are not ideal.

There is a good chance we have all bought into a mythological image of what it would mean to excel at our particular job or life role. We have idolized an idea of what we think a fantastic nurse, physician, spouse, parent, manager, friend, child, or neighbor should be. And, when we cannot ever fully attain that image—because it

M. Norvell (✉)
Johns Hopkins Hospital, Baltimore, MD, USA
e-mail: mattnorvell@jhmi.edu

does not actually exist outside of our own imagination—we deepen the feelings of failure and insufficiency because we did not attain the impossible.

And then, when we do have a little success and start to get the hang of what we are doing, for some reason we begin convincing ourselves that we are not REALLY doing that well and that if we tried a little harder, we could actually reach the level of being the fantastic image we were attempting to realize.

From a personal perspective, a complication that arises is the way my own spirituality and sense of "calling" to this work intersects with the job I have and the responsibilities I have to myself and the rest of my life. This calling might be explicitly religious or spiritual, or it might be something you feel you were meant to do. I know this is not unique to the role of hospital chaplain or even people of faith. I have had countless conversations with non-religious people who feel "called" to their work or feel that they are fulfilling an important duty. The mechanism is not as important as how we enact it. If we damage ourselves in the name of a calling or a duty to serve, we limit the scope and longevity of our service.

We all contain characteristics that can amplify the internal push to keep trying to give more and do more and be more. Using myself as an example, in the role of hospital chaplain it is easy for me to buy into the image that I need to support one more patient, comfort one more family, or check in with one more staff colleague before I go home. Realistically, the hospital is an unquenchable well of spiritual and emotional need, and it is easy to feel like I am responsible for meeting all those needs myself. It is also easy for me to feel as if I have failed if someone's needs go unmet.

I suspect I am not alone in some version of this internal dialogue: "Maybe I should go in a couple of hours early and buy coffee for that unit who has had a rough week; Maybe I could stay late to meet with that patient's son who is flying in tonight; Maybe I could learn Spanish (or Korean or Farsi) in my spare time so I can better serve our patients." All of these are wonderful interventions and would add up to being a quite fantastic chaplain. But at what cost?

Because of our desire to be the best, there is always another mountain to climb. And rather than acknowledging that we are in fact a successful mountain climber, we judge ourselves because we have not climbed all of the mountains.

I want to be clear of what I am saying because there is a good chance that as you read this there are people from the "Strive For Excellence Enforcement Team" on their way to my office to take my credentials.

I am not saying that you should do a sub-standard job. I'm not saying that you should intentionally feed your family bad food. However, I am wondering if there is an opportunity for all of us to revise the expectations we have for ourselves just a little bit. Even if it is a temporary revision. In order to be a great version of myself that is sustainable and attainable, I have to find ways to keep track of what I am doing, how I am feeling, what resources I currently have available, and my current definition of fantastic.

One of the ways I have integrated this fantasticness reduction plan is by substituting some of my agenda items that involve others with ones where I am the only attendee. For example, I prioritize reserving time and making the space to reflect on the parts of my work life that have impacted me. I pause to consider why some of the stories I am involved in stick with me.

When a patient care story repeatedly comes to mind, whether it is a good or a bad memory, I try to be curious about why it has stuck with me. Working in healthcare, we all have our own versions of dramatic and memorable stories, and I like to reflect on those that hang around with me because there was some valuable point of connection—either a connection with me or something I witnessed where the story connected with the greater world.

I find so much value in intentionally processing the impact of these important stories. Especially in the healthcare context, it is easy to sidestep the emotional, psychological, or spiritual content of a significant moment that might be encountered. There is always the next patient, the next procedure, the next meeting, the next grant application, the next pre-approval submission, the next budget justification, etc. These important work responsibilities are compounded with the expectations and responsibilities from the rest of our lives—the next student loan payment, the next family member suffering an addiction, the next potential job change, or the next volunteer soccer coaching position.

Even though the hamster wheel of tasks can be exhausting, most of the time it is easier to move on to the next agenda item and the next to-do list task than it is to spend intentional time reflecting on the wholistic impact of a particular patient, interaction, or outcome.

In my own experience, pushing forward and onward is not always a successful solution. I sometimes want to believe that the emotion will dissipate on its own and leave no residue. I want to act as if the deep spiritual, religious, or moral dissonance will somehow just make sense on its own without any work on my part. In my career so far, this approach is not one I can count on.

This personal reflective practice helps me to keep some attention focused on my total health. It helps me consider the things in my life (family, friends, colleagues, spiritual practice, community, etc.) that support and sustain me. Another benefit is this practice also helps me notice the ways those things sometimes cause me to feel disconnected from the realities of life I am currently facing.

Most of us have an activity or two we gravitate toward periodically that help us process all that we live through. Just as we all have some system of belief we use to frame how we see the world, consciously or not, we all have some sort of reflective practices we use to process the experiences we encounter. For some, it is intentionally scheduled like a worship service in a faith community or a session with a therapist. For others there are regular opportunities to reflect with colleagues, friends, partners, or family members built into the regular rhythm of life. My encouragement is that you work toward making these reflective practices intentional. Build them into your schedule just as you would your own exercise routine, grocery shopping, haircuts, and oil changes.

Some of it also requires a realignment of what fantastic looks like. It does not always equal awards and full schedules and large budgets and the adoration of your family and peers. I am coming to believe more and more that the real mark of fantastic is feeling healthy and balanced.

There is nothing inherently wrong with any of those aspirations, but my hope is that we can all make space to grade ourselves on a curve for a while. Sometimes working towards the ideal is aspirational and helps us to become better, and sometimes constantly falling short of the ideal only serves to remind us how we're not measuring up to an impossible standard.

And so, as you consider what metric you are going to use to evaluate your own fantasticness and then start the self-scoring process, I invite you to be as generous to yourself as you can. Whether it is coming from a place of professional advancement or personal life pressures, consider this: What would it be like if you started from a place of connection and sufficiency rather than from a place of insufficiency and falling short?

As the pressures we all are facing refuse to back down, I hope you can be okay not perfectly fulfilling every role you have. I hope you can see there is value in doing things as well as possible, given the current circumstances. I hope you can allow yourself the space to be a little bit less fantastic.

The Road to Aequanimitas

21

Wes Ely

As a young doctor, I hadn't understood that I could enter my patients' lives to the degree I do now, and that doing so would make me a better physician. After some particularly challenging experiences of death and loss early on, I had read Ignatius of Loyola's *Spiritual Exercises*, written in the 1500s, in which he teaches about our frequent failure as humans to attain fullness in relationships. I now understand the impact that the desire to protect my own heart had on depriving my patients of the true covenant relationship they deserve from me as their doctor.

Don't get me wrong, I had always cared for them and wanted to do my best for them as their doctor, but I was treating them as inanimate objects, in what philosopher Martin Buber describes as an "I-it" relationship. I had collected data and analyzed and classified them, seeing my patients as a set of organs to fix and a list of problems to solve. I had read and recommended Samuel Shem's novel *The House of God*, about an overworked intern learning the ropes in a hospital. Shem's narrator, while hilariously entertaining, depersonalized patients, using disparaging terms such as *Gomer* (Get Out of My Emergency Room). I saw now that I, too, had shown callous disregard for some of my patients. I had thought it innocuous to use "Gallbladder in Room 557" to consolidate both person and diagnosis, without digging any deeper. I wasn't seeing my patients as fully human. Did they know?

Now, looking back, I suspect many did. As a medical student, and during my training, I was often taught to keep a professional sense of reserve and mental distance from patients, that getting to know them too well would backfire and cause me stress if they should die. When I graduated from Tulane Medical School in 1989, my mom had given me a leatherbound copy of Dr. William Osler's "Aequanimitas," his famous address delivered to new doctors at the Pennsylvania School of Medicine exactly one hundred years earlier. Osler's words, advice derived from Aristotle, became a touchstone for me: *"Deep voice, slow speech, tight compartments, with*

21

W. Ely (✉)
Vanderbilt University and VA GRECC, Nashville, TN, USA
e-mail: wes.ely@vumc.org

the mind directed intensely on the subject at hand." I carried the quote with me every day on a handwritten card in the pocket of my white coat, as if doing so would allow me to connect directly to them both. I had used equanimity many times as a tool to pause, pull back, and process. To maintain balance and composure.

But what happens when the asset Osler was speaking of, Aequanimitas, is overused? It becomes a liability for me and my patients.

In my life, I finally opened-up with a patient named Marcus Cobb (permission to share his name and story), who had suffered from heart disease since he was a baby. With Marcus, I dove completely into our relationship in a way that Martin Buber refers to as an "I-Thou" encounter, meeting him fully within his life as a heart-lung transplant recipient. I'd been reluctant to have such depth in my relationships with patients earlier, but he and his wife Danita had persisted in developing our relationship. Taking me by the hand. And I was so glad that they did.

Marcus's heart-lung transplantation became the gift he'd always dreamed of, not only giving him more time with Danita and his children, but also the opportunity to embrace activities he'd only imagined in the past. Going for long sunset hikes in the Blue Ridge Mountains, even parachuting from helicopters. He grabbed at life with both hands. But during our monthly and, later, quarterly clinic visits, I noted with a smile that the activities that seemed to give him the most pleasure in his new life were the smaller things, such as simply throwing a football with his kids.

As we knew would happen, all good things fade, and this is most certainly true for the tenure of organs at the whim of a stubborn immune system. Several years later, I was about to give a lecture to a few hundred physicians at a medical conference in San Diego when my phone rang. It was Danita: *"Marcus is dying. He's asking for you."* Without hesitation, I apologized to the meeting organizers and rushed to the airport to catch a plane home. It was a particularly clear day, and from my window seat, I watched the canyons and lakes pass beneath us, praying all the while that I'd get there in time.

In the cab from the Nashville airport, on my way to Vanderbilt, I called Danita to ask for the room number. *"It's number five on the eighth floor … but hurry."* At the hospital, I sped to the elevators and shot out into the hallway. As I rounded the corner, through an open door I saw a crowd. I slipped into a nearly complete circle of about seven others. They'd been waiting for me. I put my hand on Marcus's shoulder, looked him in the eyes, and talked directly to him. He was the only person in the world who mattered at that moment. It had become second nature to me by then. He looked up at me and I whispered, *"Thank you,"* sauntering out of life.

Dr. E. Wesley Ely is a Professor of Medicine and Critical Care at Vanderbilt University and the Nashville VA. His writing represents his own opinion and not that of his employers. He is co-director of the Critical Illness, Brain Dysfunction, and Survivorship (CIBS) Center at www.icudelirium.org and author of **Every Deep-Drawn Breath***, a work of narrative nonfiction from which 100% net proceeds are donated into an endowment for COVID survivors and their families. Dr. Ely has no financial conflicts of interest with the topics reported in this piece. He can be found on Twitter and TikTok @WesElyMD.*

Look for the Gift

22

Ann Marie Kelly and John D. A. Kelly

It is so easy to feel worn and weary in this day and age when healthcare professionals are asked to do more and more for less and less. However, it is paramount to recognize that **how** we see the world and what happens to us will have a tremendous effect on our inner peace. Noted author Stephen Covey preached that our paradigms, or *how we see the world*, have an enormous impact on our effectiveness in life and sense of fulfillment. If one sees the world as 'cutthroat' and 'everyone for themselves' then the seeds of discontent will certainly be sown. However, if we see the Universe as friendly and benevolent, then one can begin to look for hidden gifts, even in the face of adversity (Covey 1991). This shift in adopting a perspective of *positive expectancy* can have huge dividends on both happiness and health (Milam et al. 2004).

The great Albert Einstein recognized the value of a 'healthy' paradigm. He once commented '**I think the most important question facing humanity is, 'Is the universe a friendly place?'**

Einstein indeed understood that we all have a choice in considering whatever may befall us. He added: "**Live your life as if nothing is a miracle, or everything is a miracle.**"

Thus, a fundamental question we all need to ask is, do we believe that the Universe is working for you or against you? Do you believe that adversity and even tragedies may manifest with no meaning or do they contain a gift or powerful lesson? Do you believe that life happens *to* us or *for* us?

A. M. Kelly (✉)
Dartmouth-Hitchcock Medical Center, Lebanon, NH, USA
e-mail: ann.marie.kelly@hitchcock.org

J. D. A. Kelly
Penn Perelman School of Medicine, Philadelphia, PA, USA
e-mail: john.kelly@pennmedicine.upenn.edu

Origins of a Punitive Universe

We tend to view the Universe or our Higher Power the same way as we regard our parents, especially our fathers. If we were raised by an overly critical parent who was quick to punish and seek 'retributive justice' we will tend to view the world in the same way. Similarly, an important figure in our early life, whether a teacher, coach or caregiver can influence how we perceive events. One of us (JDK) had a marine corps drill instructor as a father who was quick to levy punishment for any domestic transgression. This, coupled with the stern discipline of Franciscan nuns as elementary school teachers, forged a perspective that 'life was out to get me'. I spent many years expecting to be 'punished' for past mistakes and, indeed, this became a self-fulfilled prophecy. In essence, I was attracting negative events in my life because *I was expecting them.*

Paradigm Shift

For us, two quotes resonated within and have evoked a seismic shift in our view of the world and life's vicissitudes. The first was by the ancient philosopher Rumi, who stated '**Live life as if everything is rigged in your favor**'. Rumi, a thirteenth century Persian poet and Sufi master clearly believed in a benevolent Universe and his writings were chiefly based on love and service to others. Suffering and pain can indeed work to your favor as they are the chief drivers of personal growth. In fact, author and former Navy Seal Jocko Willink has conveyed this truth by stating "**there is no growth in the comfort zone (Willink and Babin** 2018)." Whatever misfortune that besets us holds the key to inner transformation and resiliency. From adversity we can be prompted to attain the gifts of humility, compassion, resiliency and patience.

We become humble when we accept that there are many things and events that are merely beyond *our* control. Humility manifests when we embrace and accept *what is* and develop a mindful awareness that the present moment is all we have. Pain and suffering are part of the human condition and when we humbly accept them, they begin to lose their power over us. In fact, to deny them only prolongs their negative effects on us.

Compassion is a true appreciation of the suffering of others and can be best realized when we experience suffering ourselves (Lim and DeSteno 2016). We can best understand what others feel because we have experienced *ourselves* and we can forge a unique closeness to that person. In addition, when we can truly empathize with another, we are less likely to judge them, for as the adage states—"*to understand all is to forgive all.*"

Facing life *head on* and persevering through trial will build resiliency and prepare us to better embrace future misfortune. We can decide to become more reliant on our Higher Power and gradually shed our ego—tried and true paths to inner peace. We can jettison dysfunctional traits such as perfectionism, pride, and selfishness once we recognize that they do not 'work' and suffocate joy.

Finally, patience is tempered when we embrace pain and misfortune, rather than deny it or change it, and ask, *"what can this teach me?"* or *"how can I look at life differently?"* We cannot change events, but we can change *ourselves*. Accept the pain, stay with it and ask, *"where is the gift?"*

Franciscan priest and author Richard Rohr once wrote **"God does not love us because we are good. God loves us because** *God is good.*" This notion helped us both gain a major shift in perspective as we both felt we had to earn God's love. The belief of a truly loving Higher Power who willed us into existence was immensely liberating. Many of us in medicine labor endlessly to prove our worth when, in reality, people of faith must recognize that they are *already* good enough and nothing we do or accomplish will prompt our Higher Power to love us more. When we step off the treadmill of 'constant productivity' and operate from an 'abundance mindset' (we are already good enough) we will be more inclined to base our decisions on service, not self-promotion. These are the true seeds to lasting inner peace.

We would like to share some examples in our lives where the 'friendly Universe' principle was at work:

One of us (AMK) had a very demanding track coach who was relentlessly exacting of my performance and seemed to use every opportunity he had to critique rather than affirm me. I was able to weather the storm and enjoyed a good measure of success despite the barrage of criticism. From this experience, I became much more resilient and have endured the hardships of an Orthopedic Residency with a much 'thicker skin' than I possessed earlier. In addition, I have consciously decided to be a light, not a critic, to whomever I have the privilege of teaching or coaching in my beloved vocation.

The co-author (JDK) experienced a series of misfortunes in a short period of time which ushered forth major positive change. In 1999, I was the defendant in a frivolous lawsuit (over a medication a patient did not take as directed post-surgery), my father was experiencing symptoms of advanced Parkinson's disease, my grandmother (and primary caretaker) was nearing death and I developed a serious eye infection which nearly robbed me of my vision.

This was truly a 'rock bottom' event and coerced me to adopt a radical change in my life perspectives and choices. I reexamined my values and returned to the basics of resiliency—relationships, faith, family and self-care. In addition, my 'empathy gene' and capacity to recognize suffering in others has magnified greatly and prompted me to dedicate the rest of my life promoting wellness in physicians.

The Universe does indeed conspire for our good! Be open and look for the gift to whatever befalls you and recognize that it was ordained from above!

It's all good!

References

Covey SR. The seven habits of highly effective people, vol. 30. Provo, UT: Covey Leadership Center; 1991. p. 38.

Lim D, DeSteno D. Suffering and compassion: the links among adverse life experiences, empathy, compassion, and prosocial behavior. Emotion. 2016;16(2):175–82.

Milam JE, et al. The roles of dispositional optimism and pessimism in HIV disease progression. Psychol Health. 2004;19(2):167–81.

Willink J, Babin L. The dichotomy of leadership. Macmillan Publishers Australia; 2018.

Part V

Resiliency

Abstract

For some, the term resiliency is one that should be avoided as it implies that healthcare professionals are innately responsible for their own wellbeing and that, in an ideal setting, organizations must shoulder a more comprehensive role in maintaining the wellness of their employees. While this line of thinking may represent how caring institutions interact with their employees, the reality is that this institutional support is lacking for scores of our healthcare professional colleagues and it is therefore critical that we conceive of opportunities to foster resiliency reserves that can be harnessed when adversity is encountered. There are tools that can be utilized to assess current levels of resiliency and an array of potential modalities for resiliency enhancement that include cultivating compassion, incorporating mindfulness, embracing hope, seeking balance, self-reflection, practicing self-care, and recruiting a variety of social allies. Building a resiliency reserve is important in that it does not seem necessary until it is needed and, at that point, it may make a profound impact on our ability to overcome and thrive in the face of adversity.

Keywords: Moral injury; Adversity; Optimism; Mindfulness; Compassion; Balance

Thought Questions:
1. Complete the resiliency self-assessment tool contained within the text of this chapter. How many of these questions garnered a "yes" response from you? If you answered in an affirmative way to any of these questions, consider what might be the underlying cause of your condition. Also, please consider seeking external help if any of these conditions are of such a severe nature that they are significantly impacting your life or relationships with others.
2. Make a record and date your resiliency self-assessment responses and schedule a date six and twelve months in the future to re-engage with this assessment. Make a note of what aspects seem to be improving or worsening and use that information to guide your efforts at resiliency improvement.

3. Review the resiliency blueprint. Following a review of the blueprint, are there multiple different resiliency augmenting activities that might be incorporated within a resiliency building paradigm? Are there barriers to any of these resiliency augmentation opportunities that might be overcome with a change of situation/mindset/peer-group/focus?
4. Who is on your Sh!@# list? You certainly have one, we all do. Thinking about this person and their place on your list, would you be better served by forgiving the offense/offender?
5. Think back to the last five patients that you cared for. Did your care for them demonstrate significant and noticeable compassion? Might your care for them and your satisfaction with the delivery of care have been improved through efforts to enhance the compassionate delivery of care?

Building Resiliency Reserves

23

Kristopher Schroeder

Into each life some rain must fall
But too much is falling in mine
Into each heart some tears must fall
But some day the sun will shine
Some folks can lose the blues in their hearts
But when I think of you another shower starts
Into each life some rain must fall
But too much is falling in mine
(The Ink Spots—1957)

As a healthcare professional, it can be easy to recognize some of the sources of moral injury while we are at work and in the flow of practicing what we are trained to do. First and foremost, there is an ever-increasing burden of work that greets us each day as we clock in. With each passing day, healthcare professionals are asked to do more with less—treat an increasing number of patients, treat patients with greater numbers of co-existing diseases, treat patients who are physically bigger and more apt to result in staff injuries while engaged in patient care activities, do all of this more quickly, and do so with a decreased amount of staff and funding to supply the resources needed to accomplish these tasks in a safe and efficacious manner. Patients now frequently expect the impossible—no complications, perfect outcomes, all accomplished in a pain-free and on-time manner. Even well-intentioned initiatives like those aimed at alleviating the blight of pain from society (i.e. the promotion of pain as the fifth vital sign), so shifted patient expectations that it likely contributed to the escalation of the opioid abuse crisis that we are now facing. When the realities of co-morbidities and limitations of surgical and therapeutic interventions fail to meet the unrealistic expectations of the healthcare consumer, too frequently hospitals and clinics are transformed into warzones by unsatisfied patients/families/

K. Schroeder (✉)
University of Wisconsin School of Medicine and Public Health, Madison, WI, USA
e-mail: Kmschro1@wisc.edu

clients seeking some form of retribution against those who they see as responsible for their current condition.

Simultaneously, the same amount of actual patient care work can be made more burdensome through demands imposed by electronic medical record platforms more interested in maximizing revenue streams than improving workflows for healthcare providers. Finding pertinent medical information requires that providers now assume the role of private detective and sift through endless clicks of meaningless data. These work and documentation requirements have become so onerous that medical scribes now represent one of the fastest growing segments of the healthcare workforce. In fact, 100,000 scribes are employed in the United States—this equates to one medical scribe for every ten physicians (Corby et al. 2021). In many cases, these scribes are functioning as a "Band-Aid" solution that does nothing to address the incongruence between providers, billers, and programmers.

Parallel to the stressors encountered in the work environment, healthcare workers are not immune to the outside world and the various challenges associated with living a typical life. Eventually, everyone will encounter some sort of challenge outside of work that will inevitably impact their ability to conduct themselves in the work environment. Childcare issues, aging parents, or marital strife are common sources of stress that can't help but impact our ability to do our job. Even positive life events—vacations, children's activities, and meetings with friends can become a burden if there are no margins in your life. If you have been blessed to thus far avoid feeling overwhelmed or face adversity either at or outside of work, rest assured that the rain is coming—at some point, it comes for us all. It therefore becomes paramount that we cultivate strategies to enhance our resiliency so that when we are impacted by adverse events of any kind, we are effectively shielded and able to emerge. We may not emerge unscathed, but able to continue in the fight and enhanced with the knowledge that we were able to thrive and overcome and are equipped to manage the next hurdle that we encounter.

It is important to understand resiliency and how fostering this attribute is critical to weathering adverse events. Unfortunately, the definition of adversity and its constitution is variable and depends on a variety of factors. Resiliency might be thought of as a collection of and interplay between internal (genetic traits, personal experiences, and beliefs) and external factors (social support networks and material resources). Resilience might also be thought of more abstractly as a process of preparation and adaptation that is dependent upon pre-adversity functionality and the ability to adjust following adversity. Resiliency might be more simply considered as the ability to respond to or bounce back from adversity. One published review defined resilience well as *"positive responses to adversity, trauma, tragedy, threats or any significant source of stress* (Zanatta et al. 2020)." This definition acknowledges that all healthcare professionals will experience adversity but that it is resiliency that provides the framework for a positive response to these events.

If you possess significant resiliency stores, you will be better equipped to survive and thrive in the face of adversity and overcome any obstacle, stressor, pressure, demand, or responsibility that you encounter. Resilient individuals are more flexible, more positive in their thought processes, are better at assuming responsibility, and are better able to balance the demands of home and work. If you don't possess these resiliency stores, your next patient may do something, say something, or cause some workplace event/encounter that pushes you beyond your ability to cope and threatens your ability to remain in the profession. Not being resilient creates an environment where you are vulnerable to events that are largely outside of your control.

There are a number of potential resiliency modifiers—some of which can be improved and others that are more inherent and unalterable. For example, good mental health might be considered as a key component of resiliency. Hardiness, self-efficacy, resource access, and social support might be additional resiliency modifiers. Other researchers have found that death anxiety, secondary traumatic stress, vicarious posttraumatic growth, burnout, stress, attention to feelings, self-esteem, and hope all play a role in how resiliency is manifested as a protective attribute in healthcare professionals (Rushton et al. 2015; Mehta et al. 2016; Oginska-Bulik 2018). Whatever the case, these qualities impact healthcare workers baseline levels of resiliency and ultimately how they are equipped to address adversity. There are a number of qualities that have consistently been identified as contributing to the resiliency of an individual (Jackson et al. 2007):

Qualities of the Resilient
1. Resourcefulness/access to resources
2. Self-confidence
3. Curiousness
4. Self-discipline
5. Level-headedness
6. Flexibility
7. Emotional stamina/hardiness
8. Problem-solving skills
9. Intelligence
10. Strong sense of self
11. Supportive social structure

Identifying a resiliency deficit can be a challenging proposition that requires self-reflection and, potentially, an outsider's perspective. Frazer et al. reported the following (modified for text) questionnaire to determine if there are resiliency deficits and if efforts should be made to improve a provider's current ability to confront and recover from adversity (Frazer 2019).

Resiliency Self-assessment Tool
1. Do you experience forgetfulness and/or an inability to access information that you have learned that would help you respond to adverse events?
2. Do you experience an inability to focus on individuals and the big picture of the situation?
3. Do you commonly feel overwhelmed with emotion including uncontrollable crying, outbursts of anger, or frustration?
4. Do you feel complete sadness, sorrow, depression, or despair?
5. Do you feel hopelessness or cynicism?
6. Do you feel unable to act on priorities?
7. Do you experience self-doubt regarding your ability to impact a situation effectively?
8. Do many of the issues that you encounter seem big and/or overwhelming?
9. Do you feel alone and isolated?
10. Do you feel that you have low-energy, fatigue, or exhaustion?

The authors of this text felt that one affirmative response to these questions indicated a resiliency deficit that might be addressed to improve provider well-being. If you answer *"yes"* to any of these questions, think about what that might mean and how your career might be better if you were able to truthfully answer *"no"* instead. If the answer to many of these is yes, now is the time to seek help before some unknown adverse event finds you as a vulnerable host. It cannot be understated that if you are not working to build resiliency, you are exposing yourself to vulnerabilities.

Fortunately, resiliency appears to be a modifiable skill that can be learned, developed, and strengthened over time. In addition, healthcare professional resilience is increasingly being recognized as a commodity worthy of growth. In quality studies, improving healthcare professional resilience was a factor in decreasing the incidence of burnout, decreasing stress, improving compassion, decreasing the incidence of PTSD, and improving health-related quality of life (Keeton et al. 2007; Arrogante and Aparicio-Zaldivar 2017; Thapa et al. 2021). Beyond learning the skills of resiliency, research appears to demonstrate that **now** is the time to develop and maintain a resiliency reserve. A study by Cleary et al. demonstrated that it was more efficacious to maintain resiliency than to attempt to reestablish these skills after they had waned (Cleary et al. 2014). Ideally, resiliency training would begin during professional training and be supplemented throughout our careers with updated techniques and approaches.

There are a number of things that we can all work on to improve our resiliency to ready our defenses for when we do encounter adversity. Even simple approaches such as workplace journaling may introduce a component of introspection and event framing that can impact the development of resiliency stores. We can also focus on maintenance of hope and the avoidance of hopelessness. If it seems that we are trending toward hopelessness and have lost the ability to identify positive aspects of situations; this is the time to take stock, seek help and work to readjust how we interact with the world. The fostering of optimism or hope can be manifested in the million tiny ways we react to events and situations that we encounter at work. With the little things (no break today, a patient/co-worker was rude, the coffee shop was out of sweet potato burritos), we get to practice our approach and foster our ability to remain optimistic or hopeful for when the truly bad stuff happens. It has been said that our personality and our approach to life is an average of the five people with whom we spend that most time. Imagine how amplifying your positivity and improving your outlook could impact those in your social and professional spheres and how there might be the opportunity to create a positivity feedback loop if everyone is committed to this endeavor.

We can all be trained to better evaluate our responses to external events and modulate our response to them. In one study, implementation of a cognitive behavioral therapy and positive psychology program culminated in reductions in perceived stress and an improved ability to consider other perspectives (Mehta et al. 2016). In another study, educating providers about compassion, satisfaction, compassion fatigue, vicarious trauma, self-care, resilience, and quality of life and participating in group discussions resulted in improvements in compassion, improved provider satisfaction and decreased burnout (Klein et al. 2018).

Incorporating mindfulness training through the promotion of awareness and acceptance of feelings, thoughts and sensations is an additional pathway that might lead to sustained improvements in resiliency even in the absence of ongoing resiliency building efforts. In one such mindfulness exercise training program, participants were enrolled in an 8-week program in which they attended a weekly 1-h group session where they were taught mindfulness, gentle yoga stretches, and allowed access to supplemental audio and visual training materials (Klatt et al. 2022). After 8-weeks, the participants received no further training and lost access to the supplemental audio and visual content. What is really striking about this study is that the authors were able to demonstrate significant improvements in burnout, perceived stress, and resilience that persisted 12 months following the short-term intervention. In addition, short-term work engagement was dramatically improved from baseline indicating that these mindfulness training programs have benefits not just for the employees but also tangible benefits for the employers as well.

When adverse events inevitably occur in the course of caring for patients—they can have a profound impact on the trajectory of our careers, our interactions with our colleagues and families, and our overall well-being. These events become etched in our memories, scrawled with permanent marker in a way that will visit us at night and haunt future thought processes when caring for future, similar patients. Lingering self-doubt, guilt, and depression can culminate in the second victim effect. A phenomenon where the initial event only propagates a cascade of effects on those who were associated with the adverse event and working to care for the patient. In a similar regard, our significant intelligence allows us to keep a running tally of those who have "done us dirty" in the past and belong "on our list." In some instances, these offenses might have occurred years in the past and both the offender and the offended very likely are incredibly different people from when the offense occurred. Pent up anger, frustration, dislike, and other negative feelings from events that were perpetrated by ourselves or others can have a negative impact on our own resilience and leave us less well prepared to suffer a future event or insult. Therefore, in the immortal words of Elsa, *let it go!* Dr. John Kelly wrote that *"when we accept others as they are—imperfect, flawed and struggling beings who are doing the best they can under the current conditions—we will begin to view ourselves with more compassion. When we look at others through the eyes of love, what was once irksome becomes an opportunity for empathy. In time, we will extend this same compassionate and forgiving tone to ourselves (*Kelly 2018*)."* As a small challenge—who out there might benefit from your forgiveness and what health/mental wellbeing improvements might you experience from extending that forgiveness? As a bigger challenge, what have you not forgiven yourself for and is now the time to make that happen or seek help to usher you to where that is something that you are ready to do?

If any of us thinks back to our applications to enter professional training school or obtain a job in the healthcare setting, question number one was invariably "Why are you interested in pursuing a career in medicine/dentistry/nursing/veterinary medicine/…" I can 100% guarantee that I would make money if I were to bet that anyone reading this responded with "I would like [career X] because I want to help people/animals." Deny it if you like, I don't believe you. Despite the utter lameness of our collective application responses, we were all on the right track and if we could get back to that mindset it might secure benefits for our patients and for ourselves. Compassion and the diminishing ability of healthcare providers to practice medicine with compassion (compassion fatigue) has become an area of intense interest and research. Compassion in the healthcare setting has been defined as *"the sense of satisfaction, meaning, and joy experienced from caring for patients in challenging situations (*Thapa et al. 2021*)."* The amazing thing is that practicing more compassionate medicine has benefits not only for our patients but simultaneously has demonstrated a beneficial impact on provider quality of life, satisfaction, resiliency, and retention.

Thinking about how to incorporate some of these resiliency building tools into our armamentarium of self-protective tools is an effort-dependent process. First, it requires that we are willing to start the process and ensure that we have established a resiliency reserve for when it is needed. The time to go buy a fire extinguisher is not when your house is on fire, these protections need to be readily available when they become unpredictably needed. Second, it requires that we accept there are aspects of resiliency that only we can be responsible for including our approach to adversity and our maintenance of hope. Exclusively viewing the healthcare world through rose-colored glasses may be inappropriate, as there are still many things that require improvement. However, stopping to consider our response to mundane occurrences and gauging our responses to "the little things in life" may play a substantial role in mitigating our response to future events of greater consequence. Third, what additional steps might you be able to achieve on your own to cultivate mindfulness and resilience outside of work. After you hop off the Peloton, is there an opportunity to spend 5–10 min on a yoga exercise? Instead of surfing the current Netflix offerings, is that time better spent quietly focusing on being mindful and grateful? Could we utilize our drive to work as an opportunity to engage via podcast in some mindfulness/meditation practices that might serve us better than engaging with the shock jocks or political rabble-rousers? Have we been practicing medicine in a compassionate manner, and would our applicant selves be proud of the way that we were caring for our patients and the empathy that we were displaying? Finally, how can we engage with our employers to ensure that they are a part of the process of resiliency building? It may not take a ton of effort to convince those at the helm that a small expenditure focused on resiliency building might lead to greater retention, improved morale, improved outcomes, and improved provider engagement.

One last thought with regard to resiliency is how each of us has an opportunity to contribute to the resiliency of others. One of the main drivers of this book is that too many wellness books/pundits focus solely on the resiliency/well-being of one group and view those working outside of their sphere of influence as some sort of combatant. Recognizing that each of us share a goal of caring for patients and returning home minimally scathed to then care for ourselves or our families should provide some sense of community that makes us responsible for the wellbeing of everyone. Today, tomorrow, and every day, attempt to identify opportunities to build resiliency and avoid activities that might steal from the resiliency reserves of others. Your language can have a meaningful impact on the resiliency of others. Recently published literature has highlighted how negative words can impact the brain in a way that can be similar to a physical assault (Struiksma et al. 2022). Think about how the words that you say and the thoughts that you have about yourself might be resulting in harm and a resiliency deficit in others. Challenge yourself to recognize the meaningful ways that others contribute, recognize these colleagues for the work that they do, and practice forgiveness when things don't go as perfectly as you might have hoped.

Resiliency Blueprint
1. Embrace Hope/optimism/hardiness/emotional insight
2. Cultivate compassion/identify a higher purpose
3. Incorporate mindfulness-based interventions
4. Pursue positive psychology/cognitive behavioral therapy
5. Reflect on previous experiences and responses to adversity
6. Build relationships/strengthen peer support resources
7. Aim for balance
8. Address your adversity burden
9. Recruit resiliency allies
10. Seek opportunities for autonomy and empowerment
11. Practice self-care

References

Arrogante O, Aparicio-Zaldivar E. Burnout and health among critical care professionals: the mediational role of resilience. Intensive Crit Care Nurse. 2017;42:110–5.

Cleary M, Jackson D, Hungerford CL. Mental health nursing in Australia: resilience as a means of sustaining the specialty. Issues Ment Health Nurs. 2014;35(1):33–40.

Corby S, Whittaker K, Ash JS, et al. The future of medical scribes documenting in the electronic health record: results of an expert consensus conference. BMC Med Inform Decis Mak. 2021;21:204. https://doi.org/10.1186/s12911-021-01560-4.

Frazer E. Resilience during times of change. Air Medical J. 2019;38:247.

Jackson D, Firtko A, Edenborough M. Personal resilience as a strategy for surviving and thriving in the face of workplace adversity: a literature review. J Adv Nurs. 2007;60(1):1–9.

Keeton K, Fenner DE, Johnson TRB, et al. Predictors of physician career satisfaction, work-life balance, and burnout. Obstet Gynecol. 2007;109(4):949–55.

Kelly JD. Forgiveness: a key resiliency builder. Clin Orthop Relat Res. 2018;476(2):203–4.

Klatt M, Westrick A, Bawa R, et al. Sustained resiliency building and burnout reduction for healthcare professionals via organizational sponsored mindfulness programming. Explore. 2022;18(2):179–86.

Klein CJ, Riggenbach-Hays JJ, Sollenberger LM, et al. Quality of life and compassion satisfaction in clinicians: a pilot intervention study for reducing compassion fatigue. Am J Hosp Palliat Care. 2018;35(6):882–8.

Mehta DH, Perez GK, Traeger L, et al. Building resiliency in a palliative care team: a pilot study. J Pain Symptom Manag. 2016;51(3):604–8.

Oginska-Bulik N. Secondary traumatic stress and vicarious posttraumatic growth in nurses working in palliative care–the role of psychological resilience. Adv Psychiatry Neurol. 2018;27(3):196–210.

Rushton CH, Batcheller J, Schroeder K, et al. Burnout and resilience among nurses practicing in high-intensity settings. Am J Crit Care. 2015;24(5):412–20.

Struiksma ME, De Mulder HNM, Van Berkum JJA. Do people get used to insulting language? Front Commun. 2022;7:910023. https://doi.org/10.3389/fcomm.2022.910023.

Thapa DK, Levett-Jones T, West S, et al. Burnout compassion fatigue, and resilience among healthcare professionals. Nurs Health Sci. 2021;23(3):565–9.

Zanatta F, Maffoni M, Giardini A. Resilience in palliative healthcare professionals: a systematic review. Support Care Cancer. 2020;28(3):971–8.

From Pessimism to Hope: Choreographing the Graceful Career Pivot

Ginger Templeton

From an early age, I embraced a cautiously pessimistic outlook, applying it to nearly every facet of life, including my career. I believed this subtle negativity protected me from disappointment. In reality, I was living in anticipation of the very disappointment I was trying to avoid.

I can trace this pessimistic mindset to my teen years. I told myself *"You probably aren't smart enough to graduate first in your class. Work a little harder."* I graduated high school valedictorian. *"You probably won't get that scholarship"* turned into a full ride to college. I firmly believed my acceptance to graduate school was a mistake the admissions committee would come to regret.

Cautious pessimism even seemed to help me start a family during the rigors of vet school. I very much wanted a baby, but I told myself *"We probably won't get pregnant."* We did. Twice. It wasn't until a year after vet school, a year into my career, that cautious pessimism became something more than a mindset. It became my survival mechanism. A lifeline.

On August 18, 2008, our 3-year-old daughter, Lindsay, was admitted to the pediatric emergency department at Brenner Children's Hospital with a hemoglobin of 4.5. A few days later, she was diagnosed with acute myelogenous leukemia (AML). We were given 50/50 odds that she would *"get into and stay in remission"*.

"And if she relapses?" I asked through tears. In the three-day whirlwind from emergency admission to diagnosis, I had spent hours each day with her oncologist and could easily read his expressions. The corners of his mouth tensed as his eyes glanced down and to the left. *"That … that isn't good. Survival with relapsed AML is low."*

On our fourth night in the hospital, I lay beside my sleeping daughter, IVs running into her arms, machines whirring and beeping. I was exhausted but unable

G. Templeton (✉)
Director of Clinical Resources, MOVES Mobile Veterinary Specialists, Davidson, NC, USA
e-mail: ginger@vetmoves.com

to sleep. I let my mind explore the darkest possible outcomes. I envisioned, vividly, how relapse, progression, and complications might look.

50/50 odds. I could have just as easily chosen cautious optimism.

Instead, I planned her funeral. I picked out the dress she would wear. I even chose music—Edelweiss, from her favorite movie, The Sound of Music. I suppressed sobs, trying not to wake her, desperately not wanting her to know there was anything sad, anything abnormal, about having cancer.

Despite my pessimism, not only did Lindsay get into remission, she also tolerated treatment better than predicted. She only spent a couple of days in the pediatric intermediate care unit and, shockingly to her nurses, no days in intensive care. Our nurses and doctors reminded us almost daily of how well Lindsay was doing. That this was not typical. She bounced playfully around the hospital room even as her neutrophil count dropped to zero with each round of chemo. She spiked fevers requiring cocktails of "last resort" antibiotics, yet never landed in the ICU. By round five of chemo the fact that she had not yet required a feeding tube was almost unheard of.

Over the span of 6 months, we spent 159 total days inpatient. On the last day, we met with our oncologist. I asked so many questions, all rooted in pessimism. He answered patiently. *"If she's going to relapse, it will most likely be in the next year."* Then he paused, smiling softly, *"How she's handled treatment, no major complications, no organ damage … she's been in the top 5% of kids with AML."*

My pessimistic outlook had paid off. It wouldn't catch up with me until later.

Time passed and Lindsay continued to do well. I returned to full time veterinary work. Eventually, both Lindsay and her little brother, Michael, started school. Life returned to normal, but I clung to my pessimism like a talisman. Three years later, I continued to think *"She could still relapse"* even though, statistically speaking, we were out of the woods.

Despite being several years post-cancer, life seemed to be becoming more and more challenging. Financial stressors that started with vet school student loans and continued with lost income and added expenses from cancer were worsening instead of improving. We moved in 2010 for better health insurance and job options, but were unable to sell our house. Naturally, I applied pessimism to our financial situation. *"We'll never pay off my student loans." "We'll never sell the house."*

Most of all, though, I applied pessimism to my career. *"I'm stuck in general practice. I have no options."* When I decided to go to vet school, I never intended to become a general practitioner. Jack of all trades? No thanks! Internship and residency were for me. If I was lucky, a faculty position would follow residency.

Then, very early in vet school, I found myself wanting a family. Based on my age and career plans, I believed it made more sense to start a family sooner, rather than waiting until internship, residency, or after. Lindsay was born during exam week of second year. I still had my sights set on an internship and residency. But when we decided to try for a second child early in fourth year, I knew having an infant and starting an internship would be out of the question.

I settled on the idea that I would go into general practice for a few years. We would figure out parenting, finances, and then, before too much time passed, I would return to academic life and a residency.

Cancer made that already tenuous plan impossible.

Fast-forward to 5 years post cancer. I was working full time as a small animal veterinarian, missing school plays, skipping family gatherings, swim meets, and field trips. I thought about work when I was at home and home when I was at work. I resented the owners of my veterinary clinic for not being more flexible in my scheduling, even though I didn't fully articulate what I needed. I resented my husband for not earning enough income for me to stay home or pursue another degree, even though I was the one who had taken on six figures of student loans for vet school. I resented my clients for being so demanding, for needing so much attention, even though I knew they simply loved their pets and wanted the best.

I was deeply burned out, and something needed to change. Yet, that pessimistic mindset still plagued me. I had a long list of solutions that *"would never work"*. I couldn't pursue an internship or residency—we couldn't afford it. And, deeply, I understood that the demands of an internship and residency would be impossible with my burnout and desire to spend more time with my family. Besides, I thought, who would want me when they could have an energetic new graduate without the bad habits of a general practitioner?

I considered a total career change, perhaps teaching, but I couldn't afford the pay cut. I considered an industry position but couldn't move or travel—that would be hard on the children. I had a long, pessimistic list of *"no's"*.

There was one idea on the list, though, that kept trying to break through my wall of pessimism. I found myself thinking more and more about the idea of opening a veterinary house call practice. I envisioned providing high quality preventative medicine in the low-stress environment of the patient's home. I could spend time with clients, teaching about disease prevention or management, counseling about behavior. These were aspects of veterinary medicine that I loved but rarely had enough time for in the clinic setting. And, above all, I would have schedule autonomy.

This is where the idea of hope entered my world. For most of my life, I had conflated hope with optimism. Some people have a sunny outlook. I did not. Hope and optimism were simply unavailable to me. Then I learned hope and optimism are not the same construct. As Jacqueline Mattis, PhD, MS writes in an article for *conversations.com*: "Many people confuse optimism with hope. Charles R. Snyder, author of 'The Psychology of Hope,' defined hope as the tendency to see desired goals as possible, and to approach those goals with "agency thinking," a belief that you or others have the ability to achieve the goals. He also defined hope as "pathways thinking," a focus on mapping routes and plans to achieve those goals. Optimism is different. Psychologist Charles Carver defines optimism as a general expectation that good things will happen in the future. Optimists tend to seek out the positive and, at times, deny or avoid negative information. In sum, optimism is about expecting good things; hope is about how we plan and act to achieve what we want (The Conversation 2021)."

When I learned hope is essentially optimism with a plan, I was gobsmacked. How had I never understood this nuance? True, I spent most of my life in pessimism. Yet, I always enjoyed planning. Give me a to-do list and a spreadsheet, and my heart sings.

I began planning what a house call practice could look like. What would my set up entail, how might I advertise, which vendors and distributors would I use? This planning allowed me to spend time in optimism, imagining the aspects I would enjoy: low stress handling for pets, setting my own schedule, providing high-quality care, facilitating referrals, taking time to consult with specialists when needed.

Cautious optimism began to displace the pessimism I had relished for so long. The more I planned and the more I talked to peers and mentors, the more I believed in my ability to achieve this new career path. Planning fed my tiny spark of optimism. Hope was born.

My plan was simple: I would not go into debt. I would ask the owners of my current hospital if I could continue to work for them part time while building the mobile practice. I would refer urgent cases and those requiring radiographs or anesthesia back to that hospital unless they required a specialist. I even knew a veterinarian who might want to take my position in the hospital when I was ready to leave.

My hope grew incrementally. This was not a leap from one career to the next. It was a choreographed pivot, with one foot firmly planted in my hospital. I was lucky that my practice owners agreed to the arrangement; but it was not, entirely, an accident. By planning carefully, I was able to present an understandable reason for leaving (family demands) coupled with a well-delineated strategy that benefited the hospital. Other limitations presented themselves throughout this process, but by coming back to planning and a rejection of limiting beliefs, I was able to persevere.

Willingness to pivot required optimism, but it also required a willingness to plan, a willingness to keep one foot planted on a solid foundation while the other foot explored the many potential "next steps" that might work. I firmly believe that the most graceful career pivots start by combining the secure, but less-than-ideal job, with moving toward a risky but potentially highly rewarding new venture.

My mobile practice grew quickly and before I knew it, was self-sustaining. Being a practice owner gave me schedule autonomy, which worked wonders for my burnout and desire to be more present with family. The house call format allowed high quality, patient-centered medical care with a strong element of client education. I loved those aspects.

Yet, running a practice modeled around highly committed pet owners brought its own unanticipated challenges—primarily, the need for better boundaries than I initially realized. Moreover, I still felt like a "jack of all trades, master of none" and often found myself referring cases due to lack of staff, equipment, and time, even though I had the skills and knowledge to handle them. Burnout crept back in, but this time, I had an advantage.

Having experience building a successful business fueled my confidence. I recognized that planning and intentional optimism was a secret recipe to accomplish anything I set my mind to. My husband and I climbed out of student loan debt, I set new boundaries that allowed my business to grow further, and, above all, I began to see my children's futures as bright, without the fear of cancer and other unforeseeable worries.

During this time I began to hear stories of countless others in the veterinary profession who were struggling. Each story was different: a terrible hospital environment, a major health concern, or, simply, "run of the mill" burnout. I consumed every bit of information about burnout and the distinctions from and overlap with depression that I could find. As I began to implement creative strategies for better career satisfaction, I realized others in the field could benefit from the strategies that helped me shift my mindset. I began to see a professional purpose that I had not previously imagined. Most excitingly, this new career path would allow me to focus deeply in an area that was intellectually stimulating and aligned with my values: I would help veterinarians in burnout. I would coach them during their own journey to wellbeing while helping them acquire the leadership skills to create hospital settings in which their team members could thrive.

This second career pivot required more skill acquisition than the first. I completed a certificate through the University of Tennessee Department of Social Work in Veterinary Human Support that took a considerable time commitment, spanning the better part of 2 years. This was a sister-program to their veterinary social work certificate and it both solidified knowledge I had already acquired informally and enhanced my understanding of burnout in veterinary medicine. Before this training, I recognized that many veterinarians were dissatisfied, struggling, even leaving the profession. I didn't realize, though, that approximately 50% of veterinarians and an even greater percentage of veterinary technicians met the criteria for burnout (Kipperman et al. 2017; Kogan et al. 2020) Through the certificate program, I learned of initiatives aimed at addressing this issue, the limitations (and future directions) of research in the field, and, most excitingly, I began to connect with other leaders in veterinary wellbeing and veterinary social work to explore creative paths forward.

Simultaneously, I began the process of becoming a certified executive coach through a unique, international coaching federation-affiliated program that required its students to have a minimum of a master's degree. Most of my classmates had PhDs in psychology, MDs, or Masters of Social Work. This allowed for an in-depth analysis of relevant scientific literature and also meant my many practice coaching sessions involved relevant experiences directly from the lives of high-achieving, driven individuals facing pressures similar to the veterinarians I intended to coach. This was one of the most applicable academic experiences of my life. I already knew much of the psychology literature being taught around emotional intelligence, but there was a great deal of new information from the fields of positive psychology and industrial/organizational psychology. More importantly, I learned, through repetition, to hold back, to listen, to ask probing, open-ended questions. I learned to trust my clients to arrive at their own solutions. I learned how to hold space for my clients, even when the silence was uncomfortable.

As I worked toward these certifications, I began shifting my work schedule—again keeping one foot firmly planted in the stable income of my mobile practice, while allowing the other to explore my options. The pivot into veterinary well-being and leadership coaching took longer than the transition into mobile practice. Coaching was a newer and less well-defined field than veterinary medicine. I needed to consider options, make sure I didn't leap too soon and end up falling on my face. I needed to connect with experts, mentors, even seemingly random individuals in the veterinary field to see what options might exist. I needed to be certain that, by moving into this human support field, I wasn't causing my clients harm and I wasn't crossing boundaries, attempting to provide services I was neither trained nor licensed to provide.

Networking was particularly uncomfortable; requiring me to push past shyness, introversion, and fear of judgment. Yet it was fueled by hope and, in turn, intensified my optimism. The more I connected with others, the more I came to value the wisdom and experience of others and the less I dreaded networking. I felt more confident and hopeful than I had in a long time. Yes, I was a little afraid, but I wasn't held back by that fear.

In time my love of teaching and insights into how veterinarians learn and grow combined nicely with my newly developed coaching skills to serve a wide variety of my veterinary colleagues. This second career pivot has, finally, been fully executed. My professional responsibilities vary widely but all center on ensuring veterinary professionals are flourishing. As a result, I am flourishing.

After cancer, I was profoundly unhappy. I didn't want to pivot. I wanted to leap, to escape, to have nothing to do with veterinary medicine ever again. If I had jumped from general practice to house calls without a thoughtful, well-executed pivot, I would have ended up further in debt, probably running back to a traditional brick and mortar hospital. If I had jumped from house calls to wellbeing work without a steady, deliberate pivot, including ongoing skill-acquisition, I am certain I would have failed miserably.

And yet, if I had remained standing still, on two, firmly planted feet, I would still be an overworking associate veterinarian, struggling through personal dissatisfaction and professional burnout. I would still be struggling as a jack of all trades, master of none. Now, I delight in my work. This work is greatly needed and as a veterinarian who has 15 years lived-experience in the field coupled with advanced training in coaching and veterinary human support, I can see the impact of my specialized work on a daily basis.

It may not be possible to fully anticipate each step of a career transition, but by starting with a bit of planning and the choice to focus on even a tiny spark of optimism, hope can light the way in choreographing a graceful, if a bit scary, career pivot.

References

Kipperman B, Kass P, Rishniw M. Factors that influence small animal veterinarians' opinions and actions regarding cost of care and effects of economic limitations on patient care and outcome and professional career satisfaction and burnout. J Am Vet Med Assoc. 2017;250(7):785–94.

Kogan LR, Wallace JE, Schoenfeld-Tacher R, Hellyer PW, Richards M. Veterinary technicians and occupational burnout. Front Vet Sci. 2020;7:328. https://doi.org/10.3389/fvets.2020.00328.

The Conversation. 5 strategies for cultivating hope this year. 2021. https://theconversation.com/5-strategies-for-cultivating-hope-this-year-152523. Accessed 30 Dec 2022.

Imposter Syndrome and Perfectionism: A Prescription for Exhaustion

25

Sarah M. Alber

I'd finally done it. Finally reached that goal—I was an *attending*.

I had mastered undergrad and graduated with honors and dual majors. I'd successfully completed medical school on time while also learning how to be a new parent. I'd been tough and resilient through residency, elected as Chief Resident and been given the opportunity to learn leadership skills from some of our top minds. I had completed two fellowships—Adult Cardiothoracic Anesthesiology & Anesthesiology Critical Care Medicine, and I was triple Board Certified. I'd worked so hard for over a decade, and I'd finally reached that momentous goal of finally becoming an attending.

But on my first day I stood in the operating room with propofol in hand getting ready to anesthetize my very first patient—a completely healthy elective laparoscopic cholecystectomy. And all I could think was—*Am I really ready!?*

I'd heard about Imposter Syndrome before, but never really felt it until that moment. Despite my credentials, the efforts of my teachers and mentors, all of the studying, the 24-h calls, emergent intubations and running codes (sometimes in parking garages), and years of practice I had devoted to keeping the very sickest of patients alive, here I was hesitating and questioning all of it. I felt that I had to be absolutely, 100%, perfect in every single way. Otherwise, I would be discovered as inadequate.

The propofol eventually found its way into the IV, and my first patient did great. But that feeling of uncertainty and the need for absolute perfectionism persisted. I would stay late, way after my patients were safely settled in the PACU. I would perseverate on pre-operative workups, debating whether I really needed to call the

S. M. Alber (✉)
Cardiothoracic Anesthesiology & Critical Care Medicine, Anesthesiology Critical Care Medicine Fellowship, Department of Anesthesiology, University of Colorado Anschutz, Aurora, CO, USA
e-mail: sarah.alber@cuanschutz.edu

surgical attending if I had a question or concern about a patient, or if this would be interpreted as incompetence.

My first few months attending in the ICU were even worse. I had never taken home call before, so leaving the hospital when I was solely responsible for upwards of 17 critically ill patients felt horrifying. Not wanting to seem 'weak' by asking where the call rooms were, I slept in my car a few times. I was always convinced that at any moment I would receive The Call that something was going terribly wrong.

Then, there were the non-clinical expectations of my job and I rapidly realized I had no idea what I was doing. I had entered academic medicine because I enjoy teaching, and I liked the idea of staying at a tertiary care hospital with excellent access to continuing education and innovative medicine. But suddenly I found myself with the title of Assistant Professor with no formal training in education. As comprehensive as my clinical training had been to that point, I felt completely unprepared for the non-clinical roles to which I was now assigned. Had I not lucked out and joined a practice with exceptional mentorship on this front, I imagine I would have simply drowned under the weight of uncertainty.

Then, just as I was starting to get the hang of it, a global pandemic broke out. I delivered my second child and returned to the hospital in a new world of respirators, shortages, and COVID-19 patients with fulminant respiratory failure who were video-conferencing their loved ones as they prepared to die alone in isolation. I also had my family and a newborn at home to protect, so in addition to the old stressors I now added *"don't bring a deadly disease home"* on the daily to-do list. This equated to spending all day in an N95 mask, not taking it off from entering the hospital to going home at the end of the day. I had a decontamination station set up in my car. Hard-earned breastmilk was handled with sterile technique at all possible points of contact. I showered before interacting with anyone at home. And I had hand sanitizer. So much hand sanitizer.

Despite the tragedy the COVID-19 pandemic has produced, there have been some positive sequelae. For one, my own sanity. As I sat in Zoom meetings with my critical care team, hospital leadership, national emergency webinars, or simply in conversations with my colleagues, there was a consistent theme—*"We don't know everything, and that's OK. We will learn."* I wasn't alone.

The uncertainty of fighting a new disease swept us all into a new wave of transparency, where our actions and decisions were guided from a place of beneficence and non-maleficence, rather than evidence-based guidelines and black and white protocols. We looked to each other for anecdotal insight as we awaited large-scale data to guide our management, and we learned that we must give each other grace for showing up and doing our best.

I understood, finally, that I didn't need to be perfect at all times. The effort of perfectionism was leading to exhaustion. While there are certainly moments in our day that demand perfection—inducing critically ill patients safely, intubating a difficult airway without causing harm, etc.—there are many moments when we need to embrace that "good enough" is sometimes even better. Maybe those emails don't need to be re-written and scoured for syntax errors for 20 min, when a 20 s quick reply will do. Seeking out career development opportunities created to help faculty (particularly junior faculty) navigate the complexities of academia saves time, energy, and worry that are entirely unnecessary. Not knowing an answer isn't necessarily a sign of weakness so long as you ask the follow-up questions. Ask your colleagues how a protocol was developed, ask about a surgical technique that you are unfamiliar with, and for my sake ask where the call rooms are before sleeping in your car.

None of us is the very first person to practice medicine. This has all been done, thousands of times before us. We don't all need to be "Alex the Adventurer" pioneering new paths which have already been thoroughly trodden. I spent so much time and energy worrying. I was not only exhausting myself, but I was doing a severe disservice to both my patients and my family. It would be a loss, not only to myself and my family, but to the efforts devoted by my teachers and mentors if I burnt out after only a few years.

We all probably experience Imposter Syndrome at various points of our lives. Being a good doctor (or parent, partner, friend, etc.) doesn't require us to be perfect at every moment. What's more important is to recognize our strengths and weaknesses and ask for help rather than struggling through unnecessarily in silence. I'm still working on all these things. My husband will be the first to say I still do more than a little perseverating. But I've also learned to recognize when this is helpful, and when this leads to unnecessary sleepless nights.

One Thing

26

Rory Bade

The patient is expecting you to say something. Remember to be professional but don't be too formal. Keep it casual but avoid sounding inept. Should I have worn a nicer shirt? Check your voice—it's a small room try not to be too loud. Your voice always gets really high-pitched, you're not a mouse. Talk in a normal voice. What is my normal voice? They're still waiting for you to say something. Say something!

"Hi there! My name is Rory, I'm a fourth-year medical student working with the doctor today. Is it alright if I start things off with you and the doctor will join us shortly?

***

The blessing and curse of medical school is that every single word and thought will be dissected, critiqued, and revised for four straight years. At the end of those 4 years students will graduate with a foundational medical knowledge and a dictionary of well curated words and phrases for you to use as you begin the next phase of training. Cramming all of this into a 4-year program is no small feat and no one hides the fact that this is supposed to be challenging. One advisor told me while I was interviewing: *"The next four years is not the time to get married or adopt any new pets"*. I imagine my wife, two cats, horse, and mini-horse would disagree with that stance. Regardless, like many students, I enlisted in this process because I wanted to help those in need. It was rapidly apparent that although I had the "why" figured out, I had conflated that with the "how". I needed to determine how I was going to remain committed to my education even when it got hard—what was the one thing that was motivating me?

In my second month of didactic training, I was feeling overwhelmed by my cardiology instructor's *"it's all just plumbing"* analogy. As I pondered what part of the body would be the toilet (I had compelling arguments for both the mouth and anus), a thought entered my mind that would challenge my central reason for

R. Bade (✉)
University of Wisconsin School of Medicine and Public Health, Madison, WI, USA
e-mail: rmbade@wisc.edu

becoming a doctor: what if I don't know something and I can't help someone in need? Like this plumbing analogy, my solution was simple: just know everything! The magnitude of this statement was lost on me in the moment. This goal had one significant unintended consequence: I became extremely competitive. Unfortunately, despite occasional shining moments, there was a significant gap between myself and the future neurosurgeons of America. In order to overcome this difference, I had to set lofty goals that I had no chance of achieving. In some respects, this strategy did make me "better". I learned the mechanisms of each epilepsy medication, memorized the Kreb's cycle for a third time, and could accurately draw a Wigger's diagram in less than 30 s. My understanding of medicine was better because of how competitive I had become and, by all accounts, I was succeeding at medical school. The plan worked … until it didn't.

The foundation of my strategy was that I would always have someone to compare myself to. This was not a problem in didactics but would be my undoing as I started clinical rotations. It was not until I was the only medical student on a rotation that I realized how pathologic this strategy would be when I had no one to compare myself to. Additionally, I quickly found that my competitiveness made me really good at *appearing* smart. I had learned how to avoid the unknown and could intentionally steer conversations towards areas of comfort so that no one would ever see what I didn't know. The first time I got the feedback *"you need to read more"*, I did what any self-respecting medical student would do: stuck my nose up at them and decided they had no idea what they were talking about. It wasn't until the third provider offered this feedback that I thought maybe the problem was with me. It was time to face the music. Not only did I not know things, I didn't know *a lot* of things.

So, I was at a crossroads. The knowledge gaps were piling up and I had to right the ship. I could try to be smarter than my attending, but that would be consigning myself to years of failure before I ever became triumphant. The thought of rethinking my entire strategy to surviving medical school was defeating. I had made it 2 years through the process, and it felt like I was going back to square one.

Along came my pediatrics rotation. A unique rotation in which students realize that all of their education was tailored to adults. An adult with a heart rate of 150 beats per min will set off alarm bells and sirens, whereas that heart rate is completely normal for a newborn. The pediatrics rotation makes you rethink what "normal" is. This becomes a daunting task because, as mentioned before, most of medical education is geared towards adults. I kept telling myself throughout the rotation, *"get it right the next time"*. At the time, I didn't realize that I was inadvertently shifting my extrinsic competition-based source of motivation to an intrinsic model. Over the next few weeks, I would achieve new heights as I would build on the prior day's successes and pitfalls:

Day 1: I correctly assessed every child's vitals.
Day 2: Successfully looked in a crying child's ear.
Day 3: Remembered to report medication doses by the patient's weight.
Day 4: Recognized that, sometimes, that is just how a kid poops.
Day 5: Heard the murmur my attending was talking about.

Admittedly these are not the most earth-shattering accomplishments. Nonetheless, I became incrementally more confident and a better provider each day. Through this exercise, I learned to focus my attention on personal resolve—always trying to top myself—rather than on being better than the person standing next to me.

As a fourth-year medical student, I now have the luxury to reflect on the last few years of my education and I am confident to say: I got it wrong at first. Medicine is not supposed to be a competition amongst peers but rather a collaboration for the betterment of the patient. Fueled by competition, I set goals well outside my reach and my inability to achieve them led to frustration and unhappiness. Conversely, there is always success to be had if I focused on personal resolve; whether it's beating your high score on an exam or just making a person laugh. Even when I miss the mark, I know there will always be another opportunity to do it better. Something even as simple as introducing yourself to a patient can always be done better. And every time you achieve your best, you will have a new goal to overcome.

Everyone is going to have their own challenges. For me, it was getting through and succeeding during medical school. Family, friends, and professional mentors are all there to help and support you through those challenges. Ultimately, however, it is *your* challenge and *you* need to decide how you will respond to it. Identifying your motivation is critical to achieving your goals and getting you through the lows. Jack Palance's character, Curly Washburn, in *City Slickers* talks about the secret of life and says it all comes down to *"one thing"*. Just like the secret of life, I think battling through the challenges in life and finding the one thing that will motivate you no matter what is essential. What's that one thing? For me, it was my pediatrics rotation when I discovered the effectiveness of deriving my motivation from within myself. But as Curly says *"That's what you got to figure out"*.

The Power of Coaching

27

Laura Suttin

What is coaching? The International Coaching Federation defines coaching in this way—*"… partnering with clients in a thought-provoking and creative process that inspires them to maximize their personal and professional potential. The process of coaching often unlocks previously untapped sources of imagination, productivity, and leadership* (International coaching Federation n.d.).*"*

I found coaching when I was a brand-new medical director with my organization. I was offered a coach as part of a leadership development program. I found her so incredibly helpful that, almost 10 years later, I have continued to maintain this relationship. At the time I began working with my coach, I was a newly divorced mom of a young daughter, a practicing physician, a new medical director, and a student in an executive MBA program. Not to mention, a daughter, a friend, a sister, and someone compelled to simultaneously wear many other hats! I wasn't sure how, exactly, coaching would help me, but I knew that it would—it had to!

My coach began our very first conversation by letting me know that she was in my corner. She provided a psychologically safe space for me to discuss any concerns with her. She assured confidentiality and she embodied presence with me. Through her reflections and questioning, my confidence as a multi-hyphenate (mom-physician-leader-student-etc.) expanded beyond my imagination. She empowered me to see possibilities I couldn't have seen for myself. She pushed me beyond my comfort zone—all in a caring and safe environment.

Her impact on me, and my growing desire to serve my fellow physicians, inspired me to become a certified coach. In this role, I've had the opportunity to coach a number of physicians, nurse practitioners, and physician assistants and am constantly in awe of the power and the impact of coaching on their careers and lives outside of work. I have witnessed coaching relationships that are nothing short of magical. These relationships empower clinicians with the ability to identify thoughts that are

L. Suttin (✉)
WellMed Medical Group, San Antonio, TX, USA

not serving them and reframe them into thoughts that move them forward AND align with their values.

The first time I meet with a clinician to discuss the coaching process, I ask them to set short term (1–3 month) goals. These goals serve as achievable benchmarks of progress that are an immediate source of focus and a component of my program. One physician told me that one of her goals was to feel *"done"* at the end of a long day of seeing patients. She was struggling to understand why she never felt this sense of *"doneness,"* despite her working diligently to complete all of her necessary clinical tasks. I had a hunch that she hadn't yet identified what it truly meant to be *"done for the day."* I asked her to define *"done"* and together we crafted the ideal of *"doneness"* for her to feel less guilt in the evenings and, instead, focus on the optimizing the available time with her family. Now she had something she could work towards instead of constantly feeling like she wasn't living up to her expectations. Until she had defined the term—and clearly understood what it meant—she was frustrated.

A client who is a nurse practitioner told me she wanted to finish reading a book to feel a sense of accomplishment, because (her words) *"I start things and then I don't finish them."* An intuitive hunch told me that her thought process wasn't capturing the reality of her situation. I asked her about times in her life when she HAS finished something that she started—and she named several. Given how easy it is to fail in the acknowledgement of our own achievements, I helped this client see that there were many completed accomplishments—including her medical training—for which she wasn't crediting herself. This client was suffering from a pervasive thought that wasn't serving her. This happens ALL THE TIME.

We questioned the thought and she turned it into an idea or mantra that served her better—*"I finish what I set my mind to do."* Given this shift in perspective, she left the coaching session feeling more confident and accomplished.

These are only two reflections of interactions that have played out hundreds of times in the interactions that I have had with fellow healthcare professionals. My guess is that anyone reading this book likely has had experiences or thoughts similar to those described above. Maybe not, but how would you answer the following questions?

Have you ever thought …

> *I want to (insert goal) … but I don't have the time.*
> *I wish I could pick up my hobby again.*
> *After my kids are older, I'll have time for…*
> *Everyone else has resources to do what they want to do, but not me.*

Are those thoughts serving you? NO.

How are they making you feel? GUILTY, UNPRODUCTIVE, ANXIOUS.

A good coach will pick up on those thoughts and help you to question them and reframe them into thoughts that actually change how you feel and move you in the direction you want to go.

Would the following thoughts serve you better than those presented in the previous exercise?

I'll make the time for what's important.
I can do what I want to do NOW.
I deserve to prioritize what's important to me.

How do those thoughts make you feel? WORTHY, VALUED, PRODUCTIVE.

This change in how we view our situation and our options is so powerful!

Personally, I have found that coaching has helped me in several profound and impactful ways. Nowhere is this more evident than in how I now approach aspects of control (and determining when to relinquish control) in my life. As a prime example of my struggles with order and control, my family and I recently moved into a new home. Everyone knows that the process of moving can be incredibly stressful and introduce feelings of chaos, clutter, and a complete loss of the feelings of control that I have sought to optimize in my life. I like to feel in control of my surroundings and environment and enjoy the illusion of my empowerment over aspects of my life and interactions with others. In reality, I have come to find (and gradually come to a place of acceptance) that there is so little in my life that is actually within my control.

What can I control? My behaviors, my thoughts, my attitude, my responses to people and things around me.

What can't I control? EVERYTHING ELSE!!

Feeling in control of our environment is related to feeling safe from harm. When we feel out of control, our primitive brains will often go to extreme lengths to regain some semblance of control, usually in a different area of our life.

When I was studying for my MBA, I clearly remember sitting in my comfy leather chair, curled up with a book and my dog in my lap. I knew that I needed to study for my exam the following day. My primitive brain—which can get very loud and intrusive!!—convinced me that now was the *perfect* time to clean out the refrigerator (My primitive brain won that round—I did clean out a few shelves—but my prefrontal cortex won the match and I was able to get back to studying rather quickly.)

That desire to clean (or any other procrastinating activity) when feeling anxious is the brain trying to grab onto control! It's a normal and human response and sometimes can help us process overwhelming or traumatic experiences or situations. The key is to be aware of the desire for control, to recognize it, and to have compassion for ourselves when we succumb to it (because we all will).

Coaching has increased my ability to notice my unhelpful thoughts and reframe them into thoughts that will spur me into positive action. I highly recommend anyone who is in a position of leadership—in any environment (parenthood counts!)—to reach out to a coach to discuss how coaching can help you uncover your best self. It's been a game-changer for me and has empowered me to flourish in my own life and my own career.

Reference

International coaching Federation. n.d.. www.coachingfederation.org.

My Hope

Nagina Khan

If you cannot see where you are going, ask someone who has been there before.—J Loren Norris

In 2022, I wrote a piece in the BMJ Leaders blog for International Women's Day, which was aptly titled *From a place of hope* (Khan 2022). As the Editorial Fellow of the BMJ Leader Journal I want to start this chapter by remaining hopeful about healthcare and medical leadership whilst focusing on some of the challenges faced by members of our workforce. I want to highlight the idea of 'hope' and it's role in strengthening my resilience and improving my resolve to remain in healthcare. Furthermore, I want to confirm that 'my hope' for positive change in healthcare has been a strong force that has kept me involved, committed, and working towards sustainability in my career. It has been an active choice, occasionally a difficult resolution, and an intentional decision that has allowed me to remain spirited through my own journey and career in healthcare.

It is true that the definition of hope can differ depending on an individual's perspective and how this hope is intended to be deployed. When people speak about hope as an intransitive verb it is characterized by not having or containing a direct object. Merriam-Webster defines it as: *'To cherish a desire with anticipation. To want something to happen or be true' such as hopes for a promotion, hoping for the best and I hope so.'*

Personally, I feel that for hope to remain dynamic, it is firstly and foremost immensely important to identify its link to commitment to the work we all carry out in healthcare. In addition, and for that reason I find it important for hope to possess a clarity of 'intent' that accurately reflects perhaps our emotions and feelings because they contribute to our moral character. Clarifying the notion of hope

N. Khan (✉)
Department of Psychiatry, University of Oxford,
Oxford, United Kingdom, Warneford Hospital, OX3 7JX
e-mail: nagina.khan@psych.ox.ac.uk

© The Author(s), under exclusive license to Springer Nature Switzerland AG 2023
K. M. Schroeder (ed.), *The Essential Guide to Healthcare Professional Wellness*,
https://doi.org/10.1007/978-3-031-36484-6_28

has personally allowed me to develop academically, emotionally, and has contributed to my long-term commitement in healthcare sustainability.

Whilst nurturing hope as a pathway, which can sustain commitment to my chosen career, I discovered that the centrality of hope has parallels with successful mentorship dynamics. In particular, maintaining hope as a component of commitment, clarity, and communication remains a key tenet of successful mentoring programmes.

Mentoring in Healthcare and Communication

Anything that's human is mentionable, and anything that is mentionable can be more manageable. When we can talk about our feelings, they become less overwhelming, less upsetting, and less scary. The people we trust with that important talk can help us know that we are not alone.—Fred Rogers

The above quote on communication is from Fred Rogers, a TV personality in the 1960's. I find this quotation relevant because it summarizes our discussion in this chapter by permitting us to think aloud, that the human 'self' is mentionable, it gives us clarity, and a reason for remaining committed. For me, personally, awareness of feelings represents clarity and an ability to improve communication. Upon reflection, awareness of feelings represents understanding and an ability to improve our level of compassion. This improved communication might be considered in the context of the controversy of talking about personhood. However, despite this debate, the importance of 'being a person' first and foremost in healthcare, ideally should be more highly valued and perhaps can be recognised more formally by leaders in our institutions.

The significance of mentors within healthcare teaching is well documented. It advances workforce performance and commitment, supports learning, encourages new opportunities, and nurtures interprofessional association. Mentoring should be more innovative, open to all, for all, and function to not extol a cost on the mentor or mentee. It is one tool we could use more often in healthcare to connect people who have the knowledge and expertise with those that will not often come to us for help. These potent relationships can facilitate our colleagues' ability to work through development needs and create spaces which are confidential/safe while allowing these individuals to talk about their thoughts, test out their new ideas, try again if their ideas fail and most importantly address any form of injustice, trauma, and moral injuries that are sustained in their healthcare work.

For sustainable careers, a combination of formal and informal mentors is best for helping individuals as they progress throughout their career. Careers in healthcare have been reported by most individuals as a journey with a variety of different phases. Most of my 'selfhood' has been active in preserving a component of 'hope' in my field that I developed a sense of empathetic knowledge—the connotation I then attach to 'self' is—the concept of authenticity, meaning that I behave naturally on duty in the professional domain rather than acting out a solely professional identity.

Awareness of Self for Fostering Clarity

One of the greatest gifts you can give anybody is the gift of your honest self.
   —Fred Rogers.

Despite increasingly limited institutional resources, it is vitally important that we work to instill safe spaces and strive to not suppress or separate the 'self' from our working and professional identities. Healthcare is a hierarchical environment, where many transgressions are likely to occur, to you and to others, which unfortunately you will either witness or encounter. Institutional responsibilities will cross a line with respect to your moral beliefs. It is an arena, where shame, disgust, and anger might be your only response to memories of perpetration, loss, and betrayal. Yet, when I have found myself in similar experiences, the preservation of the 'self,' has a powerful 'agency,' and has been my single most important defense. Holding onto my 'hope' and 'self' is essentially a mechanism to sustain careers in healthcare and medical research. Had this not been the centrality of my focus, maybe today, I would not be working in medical research/education or in healthcare.

You cannot teach a man anything. You can only help him discover it within himself—Galileo Galilei

I often spend a significant amount of time discussing the experiences of medical students and junior colleague during conversations whilst working on research. These students frequently chat about elements of 'self' and they often describe how studying medicine and working in healthcare separates the self from the formal curriculum. This division interested me personally and professionally through my involvement in undergraduate medical education research and membership on the Editorial Board of the BioMed Central (BMC) Medical Education Journal. Professional identity formation is frequently raised in discussions with students, suggesting to me that it is a multifactorial experience and a change process, with one anonymous student describing it as *'one of suppressing the self and adopting a profession's core values and beliefs.'*

It appears that this assimilation of professional norms fosters internal conflict for many who can not turn a blind eye to the social determinants of health that impact the individuals that they encounter. The conflicts seem more pronounced in those students who are more orientated to a social justice type of working approach and mindset. They have frequently reported that they are disappointed, discouraged and disheartened by their work experiences. These individuals have recounted to me on numerous occassions how the loss of self has caused them to feel disempowered in the process of healthcare delivery. I can relate to these experiences and, on multiple occasions throughout my career, I have felt exactly as they had in those situations that they narrated to me. In these situations/occasions, I have consistently found that the presence of mentors does make an impactful difference for me. A network of informal mentors who I could reach out to and know that they would listen, allowed me to pour some of my own sadness into a safe space. These mentors' presence and dedication to maintaining 'my hope; and validating my self provided me some relief by reinstating and validating my meaningful purpose and link to healthcare work. Reducing the cloudiness of fear and confusion. They helped me to identify and select parts of care that I could influence positively and consequently helped me to feel more empowered.

How far can we go in compromising these important factors that makeup our core self?

This is an important question to address during training and as we become established in our chosen careers. When healthcare professionals or students express a desire to leave the profession, I have often heard them recount that they have had numerous 'bad' experiences that shook their system of 'self' and fundamentally their values. At this time, most people will naturally have felt stressed and may have experienced a moral injury. Griffin et al. (2019) described moral injury as *"a distressing psychological, behavioral, social, and sometimes spiritual aftermath of exposure to an event."* For example, a moral injury could manifest following witnessing behaviors contrary to personal values and/or moral beliefs. Furthermore, the increase in burnout experienced by individuals can be further impacted by increasingly complex and fast-paced environments. Concurrent to the COVID pandemic has been a moral injury pandemic that has culminated in enhanced burnout symptomatology and decreased career satisfaction.

Healthcare institutions have never been good at navigating the relationship between developing healthcare workers' sense of 'self', including 'allying,' personal development with professional or interprofessional identities. Self or personhood has been left behind or is often a missing part of healthcare providers' identity and, in my opinion, could be part of a systemic problem in workforce retainment and sustainability. Routinely compromising intrinsic values, is depleting and taxing on the soul. More research work should be done to define how important these elements truly are and as a result implement practical ways for healthcare systems to incorporate the values of their employees into their standard operating procedures. From my personal view, this change will require intentional didactic strategies from leaders and institutions that result in healthcare professionals thinking, acting, and feeling like their 'core self' is important to the work of healthcare institutions, patient outcomes and must be given status, empowered to submerse wellbeing, and personhood with their professional identity. My research on Pay for Performance Schemes has shown that, the schemes have had the opposite impact on the motivation related to the values of our workforce. Monetary gains were not always linked to satisfaction when staff had to carry out duties that opposed their values (Khan et al. 2022).

While, we are continuously asked to behave in a professional and engaging manner in large organisations where we work and when we are on duty, we never cease to be human and are therefore vulnerable to the same healthcare system stressors as everyone else using them. What needs to be better recognized, is that healthcare as an institution might be powerful. However, those who work in these systems are susceptible to the same ills, pains, prejudice, bias (conscious or unconscious), racism, and discrimination as any person in society. Health systems work, at most levels is highly regulated, and the administrative processe's which can feel very bureaucratic and unfair. Our relationships with these systems is shaped by numerous complex elements such as clinical and non-clinical experiences, beliefs and environmental aspects that come together with personal values, principles, and responsibilities acted out as professionalism.

Fred Rogers would end his shows by saying:

> You've made this day a special day by just your being you. There's no person in the whole world like you, and I like you just the way you are.

My accumulative experiences emphasize that perseverance in a healthcare career requires institutions to not necessarily turn to new ways of thinking that serve no real purpose, or acting out to show we are 'doing' and resolving complexity inappropriately, but to have a greater spirit, to join forces, connect, and innovate with individuals at their understanding and experiences to resolve their specific context based conflict. Embracing these changes and connections made me feel a little less helpless as a healthcare provider, researcher and a South Asian female academic and furthermore I was happier to work with colleagues committed to supporting me. The kindness of colleagues has been a consistent factor that has supported my ability to sustain my career and was like a hidden gem. The idea of being mortal should be recognized, allowing the self to play an un-hidden part should be an ideal scenario in our organisations. The institutions we work for, our colleagues, and the people we care for, can move to collaboratively recognize that 'we' all have some responsibility to healthcare workforce and their ability to maintain their mental health and 'wellbeing.'

References

Griffin BJ, Purcell N, Burkman K, Litz BT, Bryan CJ, Schmitz M, et al. Moral injury: an integrative review. J Trauma Stress. 2019;32(3):350–62.

Khan N, Rudoler D, McDiarmid M, et al. A pay for performance scheme in primary care: meta-synthesis of qualitative studies on the provider experiences of the quality and outcomes framework in the UK. BMC Fam Pract. 2022;142(21). https://doi.org/10.1186/s12875-020-01208-8.

Khan N. From a place of hope by Nagina Khan—The official blog of BMJ Leader [Internet]. 2022 [cited 2022 Mar 28]. https://blogs.bmj.com/bmjleader/2022/03/08/from-a-place-of-hope-by-nagina-khan/.

Don't Clock Out

29

Joshua Paredes

"My name is Joshua and I struggle with mental illness." It was a social media post that I agonized about for hours before realizing that this post offered value by creating visibility within my community and ultimately mustering the courage to post it.

I was inspired to share this post after my dear friend and roommate, Michael Odell, left his job as a critical care nurse and took his own life on January 18, 2022. Michael was 27. After losing his mother to early dementia and deciding to end his first long-term relationship, Michael felt alone in a city far away from his loved ones, so he planned a move to San Francisco to be nearer friends.

Michael loved language from an early age. In addition to English, he learned to speak Swedish, Spanish, and Italian, traveling abroad to hone his language abilities with native speakers. He finished nursing school when he was just 20 years old and immediately started working as a CVICU nurse. He loved cooking, live music, dancing with friends, gaming, meeting new people, and spending quality time with those he loved. I can remember when he looked at me with the most excited but serious facial expression and said, *"I want to know everything about you, Joshy!"* I can remember taking a pause—I don't think anybody had ever said that to me before. We shared stories of our family lives and proudly discussed how things had changed for us both since living in Oklahoma.

On the outside, Michael seemed happy. He was sleeping more than usual, but that wasn't unusual for travel nurses who were working four 12-h shifts each week. He shared stories about the workplace dynamics that many organizations relying on so many travel nurses deal with. Looking back, some incidents he described seemed dangerously close to the lateral workplace violence that many nurses have faced and that have been documented in academic literature for years. In one instance, a

J. Paredes (✉)
San Francisco State University, San Francisco, CA, USA
e-mail: joshua.paredes@ucsf.edu

colleague called Michael *"a narc"* in front of patient, although he wouldn't have admitted it; I know this hurt his feelings.

Michael first began to battle mental illness in the early days of the COVID-19 pandemic. He described the strain that many nurses could identify with once they became the primary source of comfort for a new wave of sick patients during an isolated time. Caring for sick patients was not typically difficult for him to do because he instinctively empathized with his patients and would often feel their pain on a deeply personal level. He always put himself in his patient's shoes. Once he spoke about a patient who continued to go into lethal cardiac rhythms, necessitating their ICD to fire multiple times during his shift. He explained, *"It was like I also felt every shock; I felt awful."* Hearing him share stories, as we often would commiserate with each other about our work, I was sure his level of empathy and skillset shaped him into the world-class nurse that he was. However, the overwhelming stress of the pandemic and unprecedented rates of death became too burdensome for even the most seasoned nurse.

Michael's friends and family were shocked by his first suicide attempt in April 2020, when working in healthcare drastically changed forever. He made a post on Facebook about the first wave of COVID patients he was caring for. *"I feel for them as deep as human empathy can allow."* His death, like any suicide, has left more questions than answers. However, it also serves as cautionary tale to healthcare workers around the world. It's a warning coming at a time when we are grappling with unprecedented human suffering and death from an infectious disease that we still know little about.

Interestingly, during this time, the public has painted healthcare workers as heroes. Although the work we do often requires us to perform heroic acts, the fact remains that just like any humans, we are imperfect and fallible. In hindsight, I believe that fetishizing HCWs as heroes has been more damaging than rewarding. This idea has served as a barrier to asking for help. After all, heroes help others; they don't need help themselves.

Further, as a society, we pride ourselves on ensuring our heroes have access to the resources and care needed for their personal health and wellness. While it is important to recognize and manage our own levels of stress, burnout, and mental illness, we cannot ignore the fact that HCW's are provided few tools to do so. Even when armed with the necessary tools, we first need to correct the damaging narrative of the past to alleviate the shame and stigma around the topic of mental health and asking for help. This change must take place before true healing can occur.

Unfortunately, Michael slipped through many cracks, including known issues within the mental health system and public perception of mental illness and other issues unique to healthcare workers in the face of a global pandemic. He took all the right steps, like getting a 3 month supply of his medication before he moved and asking his therapist for a handoff to a Bay Area therapist. Once he started his new job, he indicated his desire to get back into therapy *"as soon as this 31-day waiting period is over."* However, he was defeated about finding a therapist and starting that process over again. His feelings were hurt because his prior therapist promised a warm handoff, but she had never reached back out to do this. I encouraged him to advocate for himself with the therapist. We discussed how broken our mental health system is and the stigma that we feel when asking for help. We were both mind blown by the fact that we, college-educated nurses, could face such barriers and expressed concern for those less health literate and fortunate.

Michael's death serves as a cautionary tale about the dangers of mental illness and why healthcare workers are so reluctant to admit to living with mental illness. My hope is that his death also unites healthcare workers and galvanizes us to identify the problems we face, collectively forging ahead to change the narrative. By embracing the fact that we are imperfect humans, changing our workplace culture, and demanding more from industry and national leadership, we will improve the culture and working conditions for those who struggle with mental illness, burnout, and moral distress. These actions will pave the way for meaningful waves of change to improve the lives of the estimated 970 million individuals who live with mental illness worldwide.

The struggle that healthcare workers are facing is gaining attention and momentum. The United States Office of the Surgeon General issued an advisory report on health worker burnout, citing a range of contributions and sounding the alarm on a looming staffing crisis that may impact future access to care for the wider public. In the report, Dr. Vivek Murthy declares, *"We have a moral obligation to address the long-standing crisis of burnout, exhaustion, and moral distress across the health community. We owe health workers far more than our gratitude."*

As a healthcare professional, I was relieved to see Dr. Murthy's call to action that he dedicated to the healthcare workers who died during the COVID-19 pandemic. For once, I felt like we might see actionable change desperately needed, change that could mitigate current damage and alleviate future suffering of healthcare workers. The report highlighted several focus areas, including the need to *"eliminate punitive policies for seeking mental health and substance use care."* The fact that state administrative boards can (and do) discipline or even revoke a healthcare worker's professional license for seeking mental health or substance use services simply must not be tolerated because it causes barriers and delays in accessing services.

Healthcare organizations ought to provide—and encourage the use of—more than employee assistance plans (EAPs). While EAPs are incredibly useful for the management of short-term personal issues, they are largely ineffective in treating long-term problems. Further, especially in the Bay Area, many outpatient therapists are either not accepting new patients or are private pay and do not accept health insurance. We must also acknowledge that by ignoring these needs, the aftermath of the pandemic might spark unintended parallel crises that are far-reaching and may even lead to more of a staffing crisis within the industry, ultimately impacting access to care for everyone.

Another problem the advisory report highlights is the need to transform organizational cultures. Aside from the known issues, such as lateral violence in nurses, I have often suggested that somewhere on the journey, we have lost sight of the basics that might help us withstand potentially harmful encounters. For instance, in my career, I have been part of many code situations and can only remember officially debriefing one time. This is wildly unacceptable and does nothing but contribute to the moral distress experienced by healthcare workers.

Getting to know a patient on a deeply personal level is incredible. We get to learn so many intimate details about their individual stories. When a patient we get to know on such a deep level suddenly decompensates and our attempt at resuscitation fails, it is incredibly traumatizing. Taking that trauma home with you because it was not processed at the time then begins to impact our personal lives.

In the months following Michael's death, I have had the honor of hearing dozens of stories from nurses who identify with him. One common thread is that the little things seem to add up. There are many stories about the moral injury faced when unable to provide safe care because of poor staffing situations or other inadequate resources. I can remember working at organizations without safe staffing and feeling incredibly defeated as I drove home, knowing that with appropriate resources and manpower, I might be able to actually provide the care that my patients deserve.

Since moving to California, where voters demanded safe staffing ratios, I have not experienced that feeing. But I am deeply concerned for the nurses and patients who continue to suffer unsafe working conditions. I am disgusted by the scare tactics used by organizational leaders and politicians when other hospitals and states try to adopt safe staffing guidelines. Instead, they offer vapid words of gratitude, cheap trinkets, or pizza parties. Proactive measures may seem effective in the short-term, but they serve as a distraction from the more serious issues that we face like safe staffing, appropriate PPE, and access to quality mental health services.

Because HCWs deserve more than gratitude, trinkets, and pizza parties, we must begin to advocate for ourselves and our patients like never before. We must actively work to change the culture of our organization by leading by example and demanding needed improvements.

Just as Michael would do, make your colleagues feel seen. If you know they are having a difficult time, check in with them. If able, make yourself available to listen and hold space. When workplace violence is witnessed, stop it immediately and report it. Recognize that this pandemic has provided us all with a shared experience that we can use to create meaningful and healthy bonds. Know the resources available to you and your colleagues, use them, and demand needed improvements. Above all else, remember that spreading positivity, kindness, and helping care for each other is what will carry us out of the darkness.

After the outpouring of support from the community, I was incredibly inspired and shocked by the power of a mobilized community. So, I spent a lot of time figuring out how to spin this struggle and tragedy into something positive. The answer was staring directly at me. By harnessing the power of community and the goodwill of individuals, maybe we can make the world a safer place for all of us.

After researching and recognizing that peer support and early intervention can prevent suicide, I cofounded an organization in Michael's memory that we named "Don't Clock Out." Adequate peer support communities exist for physicians dealing with the pandemic, as they have long existed for police, fire, and military personnel. That support is lacking for nurses. As we continue to build a national peer support platform, my hope is that Michael's story can serve as a reminder to every healthcare worker. "Don't Clock Out," when you leave work because you have the most important patient left to care for—yourself. If you need help, you are not alone, and there are people who want to help. We will pick up the pieces together and move forward to brighter, safer, and more sustainable healthcare careers.

Bouncing Back: A Lifetime of Resiliency

30

Nicholas McCord

The sound of air being sliced as it rushes through the strings of a racquetball racquet whistles sharply just before the "Thwack!" of the hollow blue ball is heard first from the racquet and then off the far wall. The ball is now in play. Over the course of this game that blue ball will repeatedly bounce off walls, floor, racquets, and glass from a constant barrage of strenuous, sweat filled effort until a victory is achieved. The ball will bend and flex to the point that if watched in slow motion it would appear flat, only to return to original shape before again being pressured by an outside force. This will happen over and over, and each time the ball is smashed it bounces back, retaining its shape, because that is what the ball is intended to do. This is for what the ball is made, to be resilient.

Early Childhood

First, this isn't a life story, but it is where my story of resiliency begins. I was born on a Monday in January 1982 via a crash C-section in an emergency department due to placental abruption with placenta previa at 32 weeks and 3 days gestational age. As I've been told, when removed from the womb I was cyanotic and near pulseless, weighing only 4 lbs. 3 oz., and bald. With a strong effort I was resuscitated, placed on a ventilator, and lived the first 3 months of life in a NICU incubator. It wasn't a strong start, but the little blue ball was in play.

Clearly, at this point I was too young to be any more active in my recovery than simply being cared for, but I see this as my first lesson in resiliency. If an infant begins learning at birth, then my first professors were the team of caring providers, nurses, and respiratory care practitioners giving everything they had during a

N. McCord (✉)
University of Wisconsin School of Medicine and Public Health, Madison, WI, USA
e-mail: nmccord@uwhealth.org

traumatic delivery and going through their own process of being flattened and rebounding from this trauma.

If this scene and the prolonged care in the NICU were anything like what I have experienced as a therapist in similar situations, then I know words of encouragement and determination were expressed at every step. Perhaps, we do this as an attempt to will the positive outcome into existence or to release positive energy to overcome a negative situation, or maybe as practitioners, it's our first step in dealing with the trauma of the situation. Regardless, I believe that positive energy transferred to me, and thanks to the care provided, I was able to bounce back.

To say that I was an adventurous child is a gross understatement, and now having two sons of my own I have a solid understanding of the stress I placed on my parents. Between the ages of 2–4 years old I suffered a broken leg, a partially severed (and reattached) digit of the right hand, and a broken right clavicle. Then at 5 years old, while visiting my grandfather on Christmas Eve, I tripped on loose carpeting at the top of a flight of stairs, tumbled to the bottom, and struck my head on the oak door (Thwack!). As a result, I was hospitalized with a depressed skull fracture and traumatic brain injury and remained comatose until after my mid-January birthday. Each of my prior injuries had been a challenge, but this was a true test. A test during which I would again depend on the care, encouragement, and positive energy of healthcare providers while I lay helpless.

It's interesting, what I could recall from the accident and the time surrounding it. I remembered the house in which my grandfather lived, and I remembered the toy laser guns he had gifted me. I remembered playing with those toys at the time of the accident, and I could even recall the color and nap of the carpet covering the stairs. What I could not remember when I woke up was the identity of the sobbing woman next to my bed (it was my mother, of course), or the string of visitors that would visit me in the days to follow. I could not remember my parents, my sister, or any of my friends and family, though I could recall places and things with which they were associated. This injury was unlike any other I'd had. The recovery was far more than physical, it required mental effort and engagement to recall and relearn those around me and overcoming the fear and apprehension of "new" people and places. I had to want and work toward the positive outcome, to return to my original shape. To this day I cannot tell you if it was all relearned from that point forward or if my natural memory returned as the injury healed with time. Perhaps, it's a combination of the two.

External Influence

In 1988 I watched the movie *The Karate Kid* and was instantly fascinated with martial arts. I began pestering my father and begged for months to begin learning. Eventually, I was enrolled in a local Taekwondo and Hapkido academy, not knowing the difference between Karate and Taekwondo, I was elated! Looking back, a style heavy in kicks to the head likely wasn't the best decision considering my previous injury, but things were a bit more carefree in the 1980's. Taekwondo, like any martial art, teaches physical defense against and offense toward would be attackers; and, specific to taekwondo this is achieved through blocking, punching, and kicking techniques. Aside from the physical aspects, students are expected to learn and practice the philosophies, or tenets, behind the art.

Two of those tenets, perseverance and indomitable spirit, apply directly to one's ability to be resilient. To be perseverant is to be persistent in achieving a desired outcome when challenged with adversity, and to have an indomitable spirit is to be impossible to subdue or defeat. What is resiliency if not these two ideals combined? When the little blue ball is confronted by the wall it nearly completely flattens, just as we may feel flattened, dejected, or disheartened from moving forward with our goal when challenged by a barrier. These feelings will tell us to walk away, that our goal isn't worth the effort, and that giving up is the only option. These feelings will want us to ignore the time and effort we have already expended; they will tell us we're too tired to continue. These feelings will lie to us. But once the blue ball is flattened does it simply remain that way and fall to the ground? No, it does not. It remains perseverant in its actions and indomitably regains its shape. It is unwavering and, though it bends, it is unbreakable. I trained at the academy for 12 years, learning these tenets in the Dojang three nights a week for 2–3 h a night. I applied these principles every time I was knocked down, took second place (or didn't place at all) in a tournament, or didn't pass a test, and gradually these tenets became another facet of resiliency in my daily life.

I spent a considerable amount of time at the academy, and for my efforts I achieved the rank of second Dan black belt and advanced into an instructor role at 16 years old. It was a very difficult day when I was expelled from the place that I held as dearly as my home, but at the age of 18 I left the academy because I could not reconcile my want to join the military with my master instructor's beliefs against it. And so, a new lesson in resiliency began.

Military Service

I joined the Army National Guard toward the end of my senior year of high school. A long family history of military service, pride in service to my country, applicable training for my intended career as a police officer, and a means to go to college were all contributing factors to my decision, but the prominent reason was to find a way off what I considered a dead-end track.

I began basic training at Fort Leonard Wood, MO. in June of 2000 and fell into a level of culture shock that I had never experienced, nor have I since. Once we made it through reception, where we received our haircuts, uniforms, initial vaccinations (so many needles!), and the "How to" basic training instruction we were taken by cattle truck (yes, a real cattle truck) to our respective companies, and it was everything you've heard stories about and seen in movies. It started with the "shark attack"; this is when you're greeted by several Drill Sergeants, all screaming different directives derisively, creating chaos, and starting the process of *"breaking you down, to build you up"*. It seems counterproductive to instruction but one of the key goals of basic training is to force you to find the correct path of action despite disorientation and fear when your surroundings are out of control.

This training would come into use while deployed for the U.S. invasion of Iraq. This deployment lasted from February of 2003 through June of 2004, and though time is constant in duration it felt like the longest period of my life and was a daily exercise in resiliency. My official military specialty training was as a Military Police Officer but being a member of a combat support unit, I never operated in a law-and-order capacity like one would expect of a police officer. Instead, I operated as a gunman in a three-man team, and along with two other teams and a squad leader we operated to initiate OE-254 communication relay sites, provide main supply route security, and secure the southern region of country among other missions as assigned. These operations often involved engaging oppositional forces early in the invasion and on August eighth, 2003 my worst fear was realized, the loss of a squad mate.

Each team has a specific position and role during convoy security missions. Team Alpha, to which I belonged, led the convoy ensuring forward movement continued in the event of attack. The mission started as any other had, picking up a northbound convoy before dawn and readying them for movement. Everything was moving like clockwork, we'd done these dozens upon dozens of times, after all. However, 40 min into our expected 6 h drive one of the convoy trucks suffered a breakdown. We immediately assumed defensive positions while the breakdown was assessed, and it did not take long before we were engaged by potential enemy combatants. During our response one of our vehicles was flipped, causing its gunman to be thrown from the turret and pinned by the vehicle. He would die from his injuries while laying in the desert sand.

We spent 23 h in vigil beside the steel case that held his remains. I spoke to him, and I prayed for him. I begged him for forgiveness for not being beside him. I cried then, as I am crying right now; and the tears fell silently down my face as we carried my friend, my squad mate, my brother onto a C-130, draped him with an American flag, and saluted his ultimate sacrifice.

It felt impossible to move forward. How do you move forward from this? How do you not just crumble under the weight of loss, or facing the potential of your own mortality, or the fact that you have caused the same for others and moving forward could require more? How does the blue ball rebound? The short answer is you simply must. In the theater of war, tomorrow is going to bring another mission and it will be just as dangerous. Admittedly, it is not healthy, but you must swallow those feelings down until there is time to adequately work through them. I am still working through this today. Given this, it's less surprising to see the number of veterans that develop alcohol and drug addictions, act with risk taking behaviors, or succumb to the invisible injury of mental illness and die by suicide.

Health Care

My lifetime of confrontation, trauma, and tragedy has given me a unique perspective on life, illness, and death. As a respiratory therapist, I continue to deal with the potential for death and dying daily. That's not say that I am immune to the stress and sadness that comes along with performing live saving actions, but I have had nearly two decades of therapy and building coping mechanisms to aid me as I encounter these events. One of my coping mechanisms is to teach Advanced Cardiovascular Life Support. This allows me to maintain certification and stay up to date on the best science of resuscitation while simultaneously educating others to ensure capable resuscitation teams. This helps me know that we've done the best we can during every attempt, even if our efforts are not successful.

Some of these losses take an especially hard toll. Unsuccessful pediatric resuscitation efforts carry a heavier weight of loss and sadness. The uncharacteristically early loss of life, the mechanism of injury or illness, and the defenselessness of the patient naturally contribute to this feeling. I always appreciate the catharsis of fellowship and conversation in this instance, usually preceded by a good cry. Taking the time to debrief and acknowledge the efforts of each individual, highlight the positives, and learn from what could have gone better is an important step in bouncing back from these stressful and emotionally charged situations.

It is also important to me to accept that not every resuscitative attempt is going to have a positive outcome, regardless of the effort, technique, and capability of the individual or the team.

Conclusion-Ish

This has been a truncated view of my lifetime of trauma, tragedy, and resiliency; truly, it's only a fraction of the whole story, which is longer than the requested contribution will allow and beyond the intended scope of this book.

Of note, a common theme I recognized while writing is that in each instance where I needed to dig deep and find my power of resiliency, I was never alone. Whether it was someone caring for me, encouraging me, educating me, standing beside me, or simply listening to me, I could not have recovered without my team. I am reminded of a mantra frequently repeated by my departed friend and high school theater teacher, George Harnish—*"We can do, what I cannot"*.

I'd like to say that this is the conclusion of my story of resiliency and that I will no longer require it as a survival mechanism, but I know that simply can't be the case. Adversity, tragedy, and loss are inherent in human life; resiliency is key to living it.

Mentorship

31

Elizabeth Ungerman

I perceive myself as what most millennials would call a "hot mess". As a young attending having love affairs with Cabernet Sauvignon and The Bachelor, the imposter syndrome that I have is real. Sometimes I even feel as though any resident who asks for my mentorship really needs their head examined. Despite how I view myself, I clearly must be doing something right. Or maybe, just maybe, I was surrounded by the right people at the right time that ever so perfectly steered me in the right direction knowing that I had the tenacity to thrive in situations that even Waste Management would steer clear from.

The first mentor that I ever really had was my dad. A Marine during 'Nam and a career Fire Captain, my dad is a "take no crap" kind of guy. He is a bulldozer and only has ever succumbed to the rulers of the nuns who taught him in elementary school. He is my hero and I always have tried to emulate him. One day when I was 16—as he was picking me up after my summer job as a lifeguard—we got into a deep conversation, and he gave me the single, best piece of advice that I have ever received. *"Every decision you make in life—good or bad—will have consequences"*. As a 16-year-old, this blew my mind; but I knew that he was spot on. I thought back on the decisions that I made as a kid, and the one that immediately stood out was having to choose between playing soccer or gymnastics year-round. At the time, I was looking at colleges that I could play soccer for while also focusing on medical school preparation. The college that was at the top of my list literally didn't have a gymnastics team. The college that I ended up attending would not have even made it to my list if I had chosen to pursue gymnastics. Crazy, right? My life could likely have taken a totally different trajectory.

I will say that outside of my dad (and mom of course!), my mentorship through college was pathetic all things considered. Hell, I was told by my mentor in college that I wasn't serious enough for medical school—only to find out later that she didn't get in herself and was probably just trying to discourage me like the bitter

E. Ungerman (✉)
UPMC Presbyterian, Pittsburgh, PA, USA

person that she was. But, as the feminist movement says, *"Nevertheless, she persisted."* My first real academic mentors were Drs. Jim Peterson and Linda Pearce, who welcomed me with open arms into their lab. They knew that I had no experience but was motivated, punctual, and had a great attitude. I consider them my angels in disguise when it comes to my academic successes. They taught me how to critically read and write while also showing me that even though your research fails most of the time, what you learn from it will make your next project better.

Applying to medical school was a confusing process with limited guidance. My aunt was a CRNA and tried to help me (God bless her), but she didn't know what was important for medical school. She did, however, give me the opportunity to shadow anesthesiologists at the hospital that she worked at which made me completely fall in love with the field that I practice in today. Despite being clueless on how to get where I wanted to go, my aunt provided me with the opportunity to figure out what my end goal was: Adult Cardiothoracic Anesthesiology. Navigating through medical school and the residency application process was daunting and confusing. There were so many things I would have done differently had I known but little did I realize that as I was trying to navigate blindly, I was forging my own path to the University of Pittsburgh Medical Center where I would be surrounded with a plethora of what you would call academic mentors.

I think when we hear the word "mentor" we automatically associate mentor with a professional colleague who is older, has more experience and has "been there, done that". However, our professional endeavors should not encompass our lives (in theory) and we really need to expand our thoughts on the definition of a mentor. Mentors can be anywhere—they can be family, friends, religious community associates, colleagues, neighbors, even Peloton instructors. Mentors don't even really have to be people as they can be books, nature or even a podcast. Mentors can be right in front of us when we don't even really know it, setting examples or displaying attributes that we would like to emulate. Lastly—we can't forget about ourselves. We can be our own mentors by using the things that we have learned in our lives—or even gut feelings—to guide our decisions; because, as my dad said, they all have consequences. Don't forget about yourself. It took me a long time to realize that I made it far on practical advice and having a big cheering section.

As humans we are dynamic beings—how we find mentorship and guidance will be as equally dynamic. We need to keep our eyes open, and ears peeled to make sure that we expand our idea of a mentor that is outside of the academic box. In order to be successful academically, I realize that I need to make sure that I optimize myself as a well-rounded being outside of the academic realm. I have found that holding on to tidbits of practicality and using the "street smarts" developed by my non-academic mentors has been valuable for assessing and proceeding with different facets of life. If there is a will, there is a way—even if you only have yourself. If not, you can always crack a bottle of Cab and turn on The Bachelor to regroup—I promise, it works!

Maintaining Wellness in Exceptional Circumstances

32

Vivian Ip

I have now practiced as a physician for more than 20 years. In that time, there have been countless cases and encounters that generally don't register. However, one particular evening working as a trainee anesthesiologist some 13 years ago has remained vividly stuck in my mind. Despite having been on-call for 14 h, my junior resident still had plenty of energy as she was young and eager to learn. I was the senior resident and so my role was to supervise and delegate jobs for my junior resident. Our next case was inserting a nail to fix a fractured hip in an elderly lady which was a fairly routine case for the on-call shift. My junior resident had already set off to assess the patient but returned from her assessment after only 5 min! While catching her breath, she told me that the patient did not want to speak with her because she was Chinese! I could not believe what I had heard so I almost questioned if she heard it correctly or was there any misunderstanding? I decided to go over to the ward and speak to the patient myself, only to be screamed at by the patient saying, *'No, I will not speak to anybody who is Chinese!'* I stood there and froze by the bedside in disbelief. *'This cannot be happening!'* I thought to myself. I was not particularly angry or overcome by any strong emotion since I was focused on determining the next step going forward and who might be available to provide medical care for this patient. At this particular time, there really were no other options for anesthesia care providers. The entire team was Chinese that evening: my junior resident, the senior resident, my staff anesthesiologist, as well as the orthopedic surgeon on-call, therefore, there was no alternative. I asked the nurse on the ward to speak with the patient and explain the situation. However, the patient insisted on limiting those who might provide her care and her surgery was postponed till the next day. I was too tired to think or I just put a screen up to bar any emotion coming through and carried on to my next case. Somewhat like the propaganda

V. Ip (✉)
Department of Anesthesia and Pain Medicine, University of Alberta Hospital, Edmonton, Alberta, Canada
e-mail: hip@ualberta.ca

poster: *"Keep Calm and Carry On"!* The surgeon, my junior resident and I just 'laughed' it off and pretended nothing had happened!

This encounter has been increasingly in the foreground of my memory since the COVID-19 pandemic has resulted in Asians (or those appearing to be of Asian descent) being 'targeted' and randomly assaulted. Even Asian healthcare providers who were putting their health at risk and trying to treat their patients under unprecedented circumstances were the victims of unwanted racial comments. As for myself, I have been lucky that there has not yet been any physical assault. However, I have certainly encountered racially insensitive comments, especially since the COVID-19 pandemic. One particular incident stuck in my mind when I was performing a virtual anesthesia consult and I asked the routine COVID-19 screening questions. I questioned if he had been careful with masking and hand sanitizing. He replied, *'Yea, I have been super careful and won't go to a Chinese Restaurant.'* I was not sure if he knew I was Chinese as this was a virtual consultation via telephone but I introduced myself at the beginning of the consultation with my last name being distinctly Chinese. I had all these questions in my head. Would he have said it had he known I was Chinese or did he say it knowing that I was Chinese? All the memories from 13 years ago flooded back. This time, I felt that I could not stay silent. As an Asian physician, I educated him both about the mode of transmission and public health measures for COVID-19, and that nobody wears a mask while eating no matter the ethnicity of the food, resulting in a potential higher risk of transmission.

I would like to think that most of the time, the majority of people are good-natured and do not intentionally seek to hurt others, especially when someone is attempting to administer medical attention. Prior to interviewing medical students for potential residency positions, our faculty were asked to complete a questionnaire that assessed our subconscious biases. Given my history and experiences I thought that I would be positioned to be immune to subconscious bias. However, this assessment proved how wrong I could be, and was an incredible 'eye-opener'! This self-realization helped me incorporate thoughtful and intentional efforts to ensure that any of my decisions were not affected by my subconscious bias. My take-away from this experience was that it is important for individuals to understand and have insight into our subconscious bias.

> It is not our differences that divide us. It is our inability to recognize, accept and celebrate those differences.—Audre Lorde

I always wonder how physicians cope with being racially 'attacked' by their own patients. I know that being a physician, I try to bring the focus back to patient care as this is my first and foremost priority. However, I am not a robot and I do have emotions. Perhaps in my earlier days, I tried to put up a 'Nothing-bothers-me' screen and not 'make a fuss.' This attitude likely began in my training where I did not want to let anything affect my evaluation or future path to becoming an attending anesthesiologist. However, now as an attending and someone in a leadership position, perhaps I can make a change. First of all, it is important to acknowledge discrimination on the basis of race, gender, and/or sexual orientation exists and can create problems with doctor-patient relationships, interactions with colleagues, and jeopardize patient care. At work, I have tried to initiate a policy that allows for zero tolerance of bullying or discrimination, and a robust reporting system with zero fear of retaliation. However, I understand that building these systems is a long, time-consuming process and what is truly needed is for there to be movement toward action and a start in the right direction.

About half a year into the pandemic, our institution created a newsletter to disseminate information regarding wellness, diversity, and leadership that aimed to change the culture in medicine and promote psychological safety at our workplace. There would be monthly zoom meetings inviting leaders, wellness and diversity champions, and any healthcare workers interested in wellness and diversity in the organization to join and share ideas, experiences and celebrate success. This has certainly been a welcomed initiative that has moved the needle and the emphasis on provider wellbeing in the right direction. However, much more work is required to change the system at the granular level within individual departments and ensure equal leadership and promotion opportunities. It is essential to have a diverse panel within management positions such that they can be role models and share a deep understanding of the hurdles that exist within the work environment while promoting diversity and equal opportunities. It is important to have experienced a problem in order to appreciate that it even exists before attempting to formulate effective strategies and providing tools to solve it. The same principle might be applied to mentorship relationships where any advice offered would be potentially more valuable/accessible/applicable if there is a mutual understanding between the mentor and mentee in terms of race, gender and sexual orientation. Of course, there needs to be an increased awareness of the need and advantages of diversity, as it enhances innovation and produces a wide range of knowledge, skillset, and perspectives. Many leaders are supportive and empathetic with insight into workplace inequality, however, ongoing training, especially for those in leadership positions, is required to continue recognizing possible subconscious bias, acknowledge psychosocial risk factors, and foster a positive, supportive environment which values and rewards efforts and achievement fairly. This will promote wellness, increase engagement, and enhance quality of patient care.

In terms of coping strategies for those who have experienced discrimination, resilience springs into mind. Resilience is dependent upon personality, as well as external resources and support. I find that as my career progresses, I acquire more tips and tricks about resilience. First and foremost, one has to be grateful. I am very grateful for all that I have, for example my job, my family, my friends, and my material possessions. I appreciate that my job is not the only thing that I revolve around and that my immediate family brings me great deal of joy. Whatever happens at work, when I go home, I will be greeted by my children who always look ecstatic to see me as I open the door and cannot wait to give me a hug. I am also very lucky to have an understanding husband and a great network of friends who offer support and advice whenever I need them. Self-confidence helps a great deal and it improves with an accumulation of life-experience and competence. One needs to have self-belief and tap into our own strength in order to see the problem clearly and prevent self-blame. Of course, I find positive thinking also helps to prevent catastrophization of the situation and enables me to move past the problem and focus on something that I can do or change, without feeling depressed, hopeless, or dwelling on pessimism. I find that when dealing with the aforementioned stressful situations, emotional regulation plays a key role as it enables de-escalation of the situation and facilitates reacting in a positive, constructive manner that is aligned with our core values.

Darkness cannot drive out darkness; only light can do that. Hate cannot drive out hate; only love can do that.—Martin Luther King Jr.

Some may ask if anything during my medical training could help better prepare trainees for these situations and I tend to stumble on that question. Discrimination is not a new thing to me and is something that I have encountered throughout my life. Even with experience, when these situations arise and you are part of it, it is difficult to be prepared and it will be shocking. These events might even prompt strong emotions and self-doubt. If there is anything that I would say to the young generations who are just starting their career, I would alert them to the fact that they may encounter discrimination during their career, either as a witness or as a victim, however, they should always feel comfortable in their own skin and believe in themselves. Never forget the ultimate reason for dedicating yourself to a career in the healthcare. If they should witness injustice, always stand on the side of the victim, not the bully. I would also add that **we have a duty to speak up and have zero tolerance to discrimination of any type, whether it is on the basis of ethnicity, gender, or sexual orientation.** Therefore, I feel it is important for myself to be involved in leadership positions of the organization such that my voice can be heard and changes can happen for the future generations.

Finally, always remember to care and love yourself. I do this by keeping active and spending time outside connecting with nature. Edmonton has prolonged, cold winters with sub-zero temperatures. There are weeks where the temperature can get down to −40 °C. This is where it is cold enough that it no longer matters whether you are using Celcius or Farhenheit scales. For those who don't live here, it might seem difficult to comprehend how to connect with nature in the winter at all, but the city is catered for this with hundreds of kilometers of free, groomed, cross-country ski trails. There are ski hills for downhill skiing and Edmonton is not far from the Rocky Mountains for some more adventurous ski runs. Free outdoor ice-skating is also an all-time favorite for relaxation.

In conclusion, stereotyping and discrimination are our constant companions and can be exacerbated by unprecedented circumstances such as the COVID-19 pandemic. In the healthcare setting, this line of thinking can hamper doctor-patient relationships and the wellness of healthcare workers, especially if unaddressed. Nonetheless, this condition highlights the importance in addressing diversity, or the lack of diversity in healthcare and its associated problems, which can have a negative impact on workplace wellness and patient care. There are coping strategies that might be deployed when faced with discrimination that can maintain wellness and build resilience. However, a robust policy with appropriate channels for reporting is necessary to safeguard staff/patients and create a psychologically healthy and safe workplace.

Part VI

Bouncing Back

Abstract
We are all going to fall. It is in our nature and has been a part of our collective development since we each took our first step. However, our nature is also to not let these falls define us and to rise again after each setback. Eventually, these falls start to get bigger, the heights higher, the stakes bigger and we may reach a point where recovery no longer seems likely. Whether it is an adverse patient outcome, pending litigation, substance abuse, or being targeted for bullying or physical/sexual abuse, intimidation, or assault—something will eventually penetrate our resiliency reserves and there will be a need to find new pathways that lead to wellness. In truth, it is best to plan for these knock-out punches and pre-plan to a certain extent how to climb back to where previously existed. The pathway back is going to be lined with our colleagues and the compassion, positivity, and kindness of our trench-mates might make all the difference in the world. Wellness/mental health professionals may also be significant contributors to a successful recovery. However, many of the components of a successful recovery are self-driven and rely on optimization of self-care activities, an acknowledgement of blessings, adopting an active coping style, working toward acceptance, fostering spirituality/mindfulness, and identifying opportunities for personal growth and improvement.

Keywords: Self-care; Coping; Support; Second victim; Spirituality; Mindfulness; Positivity

Thought Questions:
1. Recall a moment of profound failure in your life. How did you recover from this setback? What went well? What went poorly? If this event (or something worse) were to reoccur in your future, how might you now address this to achieve a smoother recovery?
2. Contemplate potential barriers to recovery that might impede your ability to recover in the event of adversity. Is there anything that you might be able to do now to limit the impact of these factors in the future?

3. How are you building resilience? Are there things that you can do now to enhance your future resiliency?
4. Thinking of your colleagues, are any of them currently suffering from an adverse life or clinical event? Are there opportunities to demonstrate your support for this person and aid in their recovery?

Why Do We Fall?

Kristopher Schroeder

From 2020 to 2022, healthcare professionals of all kinds were touted as heroes. Our efforts were lauded on roadside signs, we were serenaded with cheers and banging pots at changes of shift, treated to donated food, and eligible for steep discounts on everything from McDonalds to products from The North Face. Finally, it seemed that there was universal recognition for the sacrifices that everyone in healthcare made on a daily basis: the long hours, the strenuous work, and the risk of harm that we thrust upon not just ourselves but also those with whom we share a life. In this nadir of human history, healthcare professionals were elevated to new vaunted heights. However, deep in each of us was a nagging feeling that this newfound adulation and respect was not something that would last. Maybe it was the intuition of knowing that the tidal wave of backlogged cases would eventually overcome the floodgates keeping them at bay or that we knew that we would have to care for these patients with a smaller group of colleagues than we had when we started. Maybe it was just reading the tea leaves of the world and seeing that no individual or group remains at the top for long. For whatever reason, we knew that a fall was coming and it likely is related to the fact that each of us has fallen before and has developed a bit of a sixth sense ability that allows us to know not exactly when something unfortunate is coming, but at least when it feels like we are cosmically due for the next shoe to drop.

The topic of adversity and rising from the ashes is one that is steeped in legend and a recurring theme in the course of human mythology. Evaluating modern mythology, this very topic is poignantly addressed by Thomas Wayne in the film *Batman Begins*. In this film, young Bruce takes a fall and when rescued by his father is asked—*"Why do we fall, Bruce?"* A simple question, but in this case one that is steeped with lessons and motivation. The answer given to this question is *"So that we can learn to pick ourselves back up again."* The movie poignantly demonstrates

K. Schroeder (✉)
University of Wisconsin School of Medicine and Public Health, Madison, WI, USA
e-mail: Kmschro1@wisc.edu

© The Author(s), under exclusive license to Springer Nature Switzerland AG 2023
K. M. Schroeder (ed.), *The Essential Guide to Healthcare Professional Wellness*,
https://doi.org/10.1007/978-3-031-36484-6_33

that this lesson of growth through failure is one that can be easily forgotten; later in the film, Bruce is lamenting his failures in saving Gotham and is this time asked by Alfred—*"Why do we fall, sir?"* While not all of us can be billionaire playboy philanthropist superheroes, we will each find ourselves in circumstances where we have failed. Sometimes, catastrophically, publicly, shamefully, and at the hands of others. In these moments, when we feel at our lowest, there is a decision to be made that shapes who we are. Stay down or get back up. This time, hopefully with more intelligence and a better notion of how we might avoid that next savage uppercut.

What exactly it is that knocks each of us down can be incredibly difficult to predict. The people we love are best positioned to hurt us whether with malice, as might occur in the setting of marital infidelity, or through their own suffering, as might occur in the setting of illness or death. Self-harm through alcohol or drug abuse is unfortunately too common and the impact of these substances and the grip that they can have on healthcare professionals can be difficult to overstate. Pending litigation can be a constant stress companion and the merit of the litigation may be irrelevant to the anguish that it causes. Finally, adverse events in the setting of providing patient care can significantly haunt healthcare professionals for the duration of their careers. In fact, our professions' collective experience with the COVID pandemic has proven to be an effective generator of PTSD-type symptomatology for a great number working to care for the virus-afflicted sick and dying (al Falasi et al. 2021). These adverse events may be simply the result of bad luck—spin the wheel enough times and eventually you are going to land on bankrupt. However, we need to acknowledge that we are all going to make technical and mental mistakes. These mistakes might be small, as is the case when you miss on an intravenous line in a patient with enormous veins, or might be catastrophically huge, as is the case in a medication administration error. Whatever the case, the swiss cheese model is eventually going to stink for everyone and that mistake that we make dosing a medication, advancing the needle/scalpel too far, or missing a diagnosis will eventually kill someone. When these adverse events happen to your patients, hopefully they do hit you hard. Hopefully you are like Dr. Cox from the television show Scrubs who in the 2006 episode My Fallen Idol, becomes despondent following the death of three patients at his hands. In this episode, his protégé J.D. comes to the apartment of his reeling mentor and tells him *"I guess I came over here to tell you ... how proud of you I am. Not because you did the best you could for those patients, but because after twenty years of being a doctor, when things go badly, you still take it this hard. And I gotta tell you, man, I mean ... that is the kind of doctor I want to be."* Try, if you can, to avoid becoming the Fat Man from Samuel Shem's the House of God who is so dehumanized that he can only collectively acknowledge his patients as gomers (Get Out of My Emergency Room) and characterizes the height of bed by the consult that will be required when patients fall from different heights. So, feel all the feels. Rise and fall with your patients as they are cured and succumb to their illnesses and the ills that we inflict upon them. But, in this collaborative approach to healing, there needs to be a pathway to ascension and an ability to be the personification of a healthcare phoenix that allows you to continue in your career.

In many cases, the key to recovery and resiliency is proactively building up reserves, pathways, infrastructure, and/or coping mechanisms that will serve as buoying mechanisms following the adverse event. However, there may be times when these resiliency efforts alone prove insufficient in avoiding a catastrophic tailspin. Whether there is one tremendously horrendous inciting event or multiple small events and situations that coalesce to knock your ass to the mat, there are times when the idea of rising again may seem incongruent with your current situation and navigating a path out of a particular quagmire may seem impossible.

In the healthcare setting, the idea of the second victim is one that has recently gained traction as a mechanism to recognize that adverse events in a healthcare setting have a ripple effect that do not end only with the afflicted patient and their family. After being first described, the idea of the second victim was well-defined as "a health care provider involved in an unanticipated adverse patient event, medical error and/or a patient related-injury who becomes victimized in the sense that the provider is traumatized by the event. Frequently, second victims feel personally responsible for the unexpected patient outcomes and feel as though they have failed their patient, and feel doubts about their clinical skills and knowledge base (Scott et al. 2009, 2010)." Following an adverse event, healthcare workers can encounter significant feelings of guilt, incompetence, or inadequacy. In some cases, it may have been a medical error that resulted in patient harm but, in many cases, even being in proximity to an adverse event or intensively emotional situation can result in an emotional tsunami that can wash over all other aspects of a person's life. Unfortunately, this second victim phenomenon is not a unique or isolated occurrence. In one study of all staff members at a large healthcare system, nearly one in seven staff members reported that they had experienced a patient safety event within the past year that negatively impacted them through feelings of anxiety, depression, or introspective concerns and that these workers were unable to effectively perform their job. For the staff members at the institution of interest, assistance from the institution itself was not tremendously forthcoming and 68% reported that they did not receive any support from the institution that addressed their wellbeing following the event (Susan and Scott 2011). This prevalence demands that there is a system in place for our colleagues to ensure their safety and promote their well-being. In a survey of over 900 practitioners, effective coping mechanisms were identified as debriefing with the involved medical team, talking with colleagues, and discussing the outcome with patients and their families (Kaur et al. 2019). Additional effective strategies have included increasing institutional peer support infrastructure and ensuring that this support is available 24/7, creating structured sessions for healthcare professionals involved in adverse events, encouraging leaders within the organization to be forthcoming with their own history of adverse events and share their strategies for navigation of these situations, and proactively working to treat burnout and promote empathy. Other groups have advocated providing confidential forums where adverse events can be discussed and hosting events that describe the second victim phenomenon so that there is a collective understanding of what it is and how it will be addressed. What needs to be remembered is that these colleagues should not be isolated and following an adverse event is the time to rally to support our colleagues and not the time to leave them in isolation (Seys et al. 2013). One point worth mentioning, however, is that there is an evolving sentiment that pushes back against the idea of healthcare professionals as victims in the setting of medical errors or adverse events. Those opposed to this idea feel that victim labeling introduces a passive quality to the nature of these events and an inappropriate absolvement of guilt. Those opposed to healthcare professional victim labeling may have witnessed, often in friends and family, how medical errors have the potential to elicit catastrophic harm (Clarkson et al. 2019). Unfortunately, this approach assumes that the victim labeling of one group somehow diminishes the victim status or tragedy of another. This would be akin to two people emerging from a rainstorm and stating that the soaked status of one of the two diminishes that of the other. While what occasionally happens to our patients and their families is undeniably tragic, so too is the impact of these events on our colleagues. To deny the impact of these adverse medical events on healthcare workers ignores recently published research demonstrating that the risk of suicide in bedside nurses is up to 58% higher than the general US population and that lack of support following adverse events is a leading cause of this tragic event (Davidson et al. 2019).

A recently touted strategy for the improvement of healthcare worker resiliency suggests that the solution is much simpler than what we have made it out to be. Simply, there is a collective need in healthcare to focus on addressing the way that we treat each other and move toward a paradigm where we treat each other with forgiveness, thoughtfulness, and kindness. Like an insidious virus, emotions and routine behaviors can propagate and spread within an organization. Rudeness, toxicity, abuse, and bullying become perpetuated as healthcare workers retreat into their limited silos or tribes and seek to assign blame for their current condition on those outside of that limited group instead of recognizing the system as the source of most insults. Unfortunately, this approach can leave individuals as sole inhabitants of islands of toxicity and without effective support when adversity emerges. The healthcare industry has been identified as one of the least civil industries and one where unkind and disruptive behavior is too frequently the norm (Protomag n.d.). A 2022 survey of 1500 physicians found that 62% of physicians had witnessed colleagues acting inappropriately; this rate of inappropriate behavior increased 6% from 2021, and that the average number of witnessed inappropriate events had also increased. However, it seems that physicians may not be outstanding at identifying their own bad behavior as this same study found that only 13% identified themselves as a contributor to poor behavior in the past year (McKenna 2022). Imagine if all healthcare professionals sought to consciously pursue opportunities to bolster their colleagues, approach conflict situations from a position of attempted understanding, and identify opportunities to spread kindness. This approach would very likely lead to an expansion of networks and a healthcare environment more conducive to supporting colleagues in times of need.

In every superhero arc, there is inevitably a moment where it appears that all is lost and that the villain will prevail. As healthcare professionals, it is important to anticipate this fall and consider the Japanese proverb *"Nana korobi ya oki"* which means *"fall down seven times, get up eight."* However, Rocky Balboa offered some amazing advice when he extolled—*"Let me tell you something you already know. The world ain't all sunshine and rainbows. It's a very mean and nasty place and I don't care how tough you are it will beat you to your knees and keep you there permanently if you let it. You, me, or nobody is going to hit as hard as life. But it ain't about how hard ya hit. It's about how hard you can get hit and keep moving forward. How much you can take and keep moving forward. That's how winning is done!"* These phrases provide tremendous inspiration to get up, move forward, and move past the event that resulted in our ass being knocked to the mat. However, the process is not always so easy and getting back up from the ground requires a number of steps. How you get up is likely going to be an individual process. However, there are some processes that might lead to a greater chance of a successful rebound.

Blueprint for Bouncing Back:
1. Engage your support network
2. Consider seeking professional advice/care
3. Optimize self-care activities
4. Seek out opportunities for positivity
5. Acknowledge blessings
6. Adopt an active coping style
7. Work toward acceptance
8. Foster spirituality/mindfulness
9. Seek inspiration
10. Identify opportunities for growth and improvement

For the small workplace jabs, it may only require a short period of introspection and a focus on aspects of self-care to realize effective improvements. However, there are going to be some events that cannot be outrun and for which no amount of exercise, rest, or clean eating can erase the stain on our psyches. In these situations, engaging the help of others becomes critical. Even the mightiest among us will occasionally require assistance from another and it needs to become more normalized and accepted for us to seek opportunities to engage with these resources.

You are all heroes—and despite the adversity that you may encounter *"You are much stronger than you think you are. Trust me."* Superman.

References

al Falasi B, al Mazrouei M, al Ali M, et al. Prevalence and determinants of immediate and long-term PTSD consequences of coronavirus-related (CoV-1 and CoV-2) pandemics among healthcare professionals: a systematic review and meta-analysis. Int J Environ Res Public Health. 2021;18(4):2182. https://doi.org/10.3390/ijerph18042182.

Clarkson MD, Haskell H, Hemmelgarn C, et al. Abandon the term "second victim.". BMJ. 2019;364:l1233. https://doi.org/10.1136/bmj.l1233.

Davidson JE, Proudfoot J, Lee K, Zisook S. Nurse suicide in the United States: analysis of the Center for Disease Control 2014 National Violent Death Reporting System dataset. Arch Psychiatr Nurs. 2019;33:16–21.

Kaur AP, Levinson AT, Monteiro JF, et al. The impact of errors on healthcare professionals in the critical care setting. J Crit Care. 2019;52:16–21.

Jon McKenna. Physicians behaving badly: stress and hardship trigger misconduct. 2022. https://www.medscape.com/slideshow/2022-physicians-misbehaving-6015583?faf=1#. Accessed 4 Dec 2022.

Protomag. Be nice. n.d.. https://protomag.com/policy/be-nice. Accessed 4 Dec 2022.

Scott SD, Hirschinger LE, Cox KR, et al. The natural history of recovery for the healthcare provider "second victim" after adverse patient events. Qual Saf Health Care. 2009;18(5):325–30.

Scott SD, Hirschinger LE, Cox KR, et al. Caring for our own: deploying a systemwide second victim rapid response team. Jt Comm J Qual Patient Saf. 2010;36(5):233–40.

Seys D, Scott S, Wu A, et al. Supporting involved health care professionals (second victims) following an adverse health event: a literature review. Int J Nurs Stud. 2013;50(5):678–87.

Susan D, Scott RN. The second victim phenomenon: a harsh reality of health care professions. 2011. https://psnet.ahrq.gov/perspective/second-victim-phenomenon-harsh-reality-healthcare-professions. Accessed 1 Dec 2022.

Road to Recovery

34

Jillian Rigert

When I developed suicidal ideation as an oral and maxillofacial surgery resident in 2014, I thought I was the only one.

I thought I was weak.

I thought that my inability to function in super-human conditions meant that I was sub-human.

My negative self-talk was accentuated during long periods of sleep deprivation and, though I am not a mental health professional, I do not recommend doing what I did—isolating due to feelings of inadequacy and playing a broken record of negative beliefs about myself which did not pave the path towards healing.

By 2017, I had to jump off the merry-go-round. Fortunately, I jumped towards rest and ultimately writing —both of which have been essential steps in the healing journey. However, the choice was not clear. When sleep deprived and desperate for relief, it can be hard to think clearly.

Thus, if you are there, now, I want you to know you are not alone and healing is possible. In 2017—it took one person to tell me that I was not alone to step back and realize I was not broken. Often, we are humans working in a system made for robots—wondering why we are becoming ill. We are humans. Not robots. We need a system made for humans.

While we work to improve our environments, we can start healing immediately. First—provide yourself permission to seek what you need in this moment. I needed to rest, yet it took me 5 years to rest after I transferred residencies. The delay was a result of my resistance to sitting in the discomfort of my own thoughts. I threw myself into long hours at work to distract myself from feelings of inadequacy which only prolonged the suffering. Relate?

Writing has been essential throughout the journey. Re-reading journals I had in 2014–2017 revealed to me just how dark my thoughts were becoming and helped me to connect that long periods of sleep deprivation were a common thread in

J. Rigert (✉)
Houston, TX, USA

periods of mental health decline. There are several communities where healthcare professionals share their writing—these communities have been core to my deeper healing, and I invite you to find your communities if you have not already.

Previously silenced by the guilt and shame of not being enough and feeling like a "quitter" after leaving surgery—sharing my writing about my journey helped connect me to people who resonated deeply. At various stages in our healing, we came together with diverse forms of solutions. These communities provided me the opportunity to finally give myself permission—permission to pivot and permission to let go of all the guilt, shame, and feelings of never being enough.

And through being vulnerable, sharing my innermost insecurities and shining light on my darkest thoughts, I realized that—when we are authentically ourselves—we open up the opportunity to invite people into our lives who resonate with our stories and need to heal, too.

We are strong. Stronger together.

And nothing in your career is more important than your life. Nothing.

Please seek immediate help if you are experiencing thoughts of suicide. Help is available, healing is possible and your life matters. You matter, and you are loved.

Sometimes Caregivers Need Professional Help Too

35

Brooke Anderson

Movies about overcoming adversity often have a pivotal scene where the main character has the realization that their life is about to be forever altered. For me, that moment occurred on September 11, 2001. The day our nation was attacked, and the military started down the path towards war.

A little about my back story. I have always loved new experiences and learning about other cultures. I was fortunate that my family often hosted exchange students from other countries and cultures, which fueled my love of travel and adventure. As a senior in high school, I became a rotary exchange student to Brazil, and then in college I spent two summers living in Panama. Once I started traveling, I was hooked. So, when I started working at the local Veteran's Affairs Hospital after graduating from nursing school, I loved hearing about all the travel my patients experienced in the military. Soon after starting at the VA, I submitted an online form to contact a recruiter on a whim. The next week, I was in the recruiter's office signing paperwork to enlist as an officer in the United States Air Force. I started basic training on 9/2/2001 in Montgomery, Alabama. During my second week of basic training, 9/11 happened and my life was forever altered, but not in the way that I expected.

In February 2003, I was notified that in less than 2 weeks' time I was deploying as part of a field hospital to the Middle East. I was a bundle of emotions that ranged from excited to terrified, and I also felt a strong sense that this was why I had been drawn to the military in the first place. Yes, I love to travel, but I also felt a strong sense of duty and the desire to make sure our wounded troops made it back home to their loved ones. I felt like I had finally found my calling in life, and I was ready.

In March 2003, we reached the Middle East, and rapidly set up our tent hospital. We invaded Iraq on March 19, 2003, and the casualties started coming in. Although I had a good solid foundation as a nurse, nothing prepared me for what I was about

B. Anderson (✉)
University of Wisconsin School of Medicine and Public Health, Madison, WI, USA
e-mail: brooke.anderson@ctri.wisc.edu

© The Author(s), under exclusive license to Springer Nature Switzerland AG 2023
K. M. Schroeder (ed.), *The Essential Guide to Healthcare Professional Wellness*,
https://doi.org/10.1007/978-3-031-36484-6_35

to see. My colleagues and I had to learn a lot on the job, with limited resources and support. In the beginning, I worried every day that my lack of knowledge and training was going to harm someone, but over time, I realized I knew more than I thought I did, and my confidence grew.

To escape the hospital and relax, I befriended several of the Army medical personnel. We would frequently watch movies, play cards, and just hang out. On March 21, 2003, they threw a party to celebrate the Afghan New Year. Although it started off as a fun time with friends, it ended when a "friend" betrayed my trust and would not take *"no"* for an answer. That night changed my life forever. I considered reporting what happened but feared that I would be the one who was blamed, so I kept my mouth shut for many, many years and pretended it never happened.

Following my deployment, upon return to my home base, I started to develop numerous health problems including frequent headaches, constant nausea, joint pains, and severe insomnia. I was tested for many things, and everything came back negative. The medical professionals told me to lose weight and started me on medication for depression. My supervisor and my colleagues started hinting that I was lazy and just did not want to work. Considering I was always the first person to volunteer for everything prior to my deployment, it was like a kick in the gut to be judged, and to feel like there was no support from those around me. My last year in the military was one of the most stressful of my life. Because they could not find anything wrong with me, I had to continue working 12-h shifts and I was not allowed to call in sick, despite there being days I was so tired that I was not only a danger to myself, but to others. On occasion I was so tired after work I would have to pull over on the side of the road to close my eyes before I could continue home. I was terrified of what would happen when I ultimately separated from the military. All my training was as an intensive care unit nurse, but I feared my mind and body could not handle the stress of 12-h rotating shifts. To cope with the stress of everything I started drinking and going out, sometimes to excess. It was easier to forget things when I was surrounded by people, and alcohol made me feel more relaxed.

After I separated from the military in September 2005, I moved back to my home state. Thinking it would be easier on my body than being a staff nurse, I accepted a position as a nurse manager for a hospital that was about to open. My problems with headaches, nausea, insomnia, and chronic pain worsened. I underwent test after test, trying to figure out what was wrong. Although I cut back on alcohol, I started working 60–80 h a week. When I was not working, I stayed as busy as possible. At the time I did not realize it, but I had replaced a reliance on alcohol with working all the time to keep myself from thinking and feeling. My relationships fell apart and I struggled every day. At one point, I started having memory problems and high blood pressure. I was afraid I was going to have a heart attack or a nervous breakdown before age 30. Given the large amount of money I was spending on medical costs, I finally decided to apply for military disability compensation.

The night before my compensation and pension exam, I had a lengthy conversation with my mother about which conditions I was applying for. I was requesting a review of my migraines, irritable bowel syndrome, and fibromyalgia. My mother asked why I was not also applying for PTSD. I remember laughing. She pointed out that I came back after my first deployment and put everything in a box, and never spoke of it again. That night as I lay awake thinking back on my deployment, I was hit by wave after wave of emotions. All the memories I spent years trying to suppress came back to me, and I had one of the worst panic attacks of my life. When I spoke to the compensation and pension examiner, it was the first time I admitted the "incident" out loud. However, being a healthcare professional, even after sharing what happened, I still believed I had things under control, and I continued to deny the need for professional help.

In January 2011, my husband and I welcomed our first child. Being a mother changed my life in many ways, many of them positive. However, looking back, I can tell the increased stress of pregnancy and motherhood exacerbated my PTSD. I started sleeping with pillows surrounding me so that my husband would not accidentally touch me while I slept. I used ear plugs and a white noise machine to sleep, because I was constantly vigilant about noises, even in my sleep. I hated being touched in any way, including something as simple as a hug. It finally came to a head 1 day while I was sitting on the floor. My almost 1 year-old ran up behind me and threw his arms around me, and I responded as though I were being attacked. Realizing that I could misconstrue my child's affection as a threat was the wake-up call that helped me see I needed help. It took me 9 years from "the incident" to finally come to this realization.

I was very fortunate that the hospital department I was working for at the time emphasized the importance of family and self-care. They worked to arrange my clinical schedule around weekly behavioral therapy appointments and allowed me time off when I was too emotionally spent to work. I went through several months of weekly prolonged exposure therapy before I was able to speak about what happened to me without going into a panic. They also worked with me on cognitive behavioral therapy, to learn how to cope with many of the other traumas I experienced during my military service. I was finally starting to feel happy and whole again, and thought I was finally learning to let go of the past.

Things were better for several years, and I transitioned to a different department in the hospital. After the birth of my second child, many of my physical symptoms worsened again. I started having regular headaches, nausea, and insomnia. Unfortunately, at that time, I still had not learned that many of my physical symptoms were triggered by a combination of PTSD and stress. My new supervisor was not as understanding about my health problems, and strictly followed the institutions' absence policy. As soon as I accumulated more than three unplanned absences in a 12-week rolling calendar, I was placed in the disciplinary process. The fear of losing my job made everything worse, and the toll of these stressors started to impact my marriage and my friendships.

When a part-time position in our hospital opened, I jumped at it, hoping that the decrease in hours would help with my stress level. Although that was not the case, I did learn something incredibly valuable while in that job. I started to learn more about the mind-body connection and how PTSD is often manifested through physical symptoms like headaches, nausea, and insomnia, and is worsened by stress. Despite knowing about PTSD, the various symptoms, and the ways to treat it, when it came to my personal experience, I was blind. I also learned that my use of alcohol, and then work, to escape my thoughts were very common coping methods. I got back into therapy and agreed to a trial of an anti-depressant. I cut back on work hours and started focusing more on myself and my family, as well as developing new, more positive, coping methods. Music and dance became my new passion. Things were not perfect, but over time, my symptoms continued to improve.

I have learned that living with PTSD is a journey. When my stress level is low, and my mood is good, my PTSD symptoms are manageable. However, when something stressful occurs, like the death of my best friend, or a triggering event happens, like the invasion of Ukraine, my symptoms worsen. I have also learned that although I am a healthcare professional, I will need professional help off and on throughout my life, and there is no shame in that. Everyone needs extra help sometimes.

I hope that by sharing my experience, other survivors realize it is not only okay, but essential, to ask for professional help when you need it, even though, as a healthcare provider, you feel you "should" be able to handle it. I also hope that colleagues, supervisors, and even friends, learn to recognize that physical symptoms may be the manifestation of mental health problems. Excessive use of alcohol or trying to keep constantly busy are also clues that someone may be trying to escape from something. Rather than criticize people as being lazy, please consider showing empathy and support.

It is incredibly important for supervisors to be aware that it is your responsibility to notify employees about resources available to them and their rights under the Family Medical Leave Act (FMLA) if you have reason to believe their absence may be covered. By alerting employees like me to available resources and accommodations, you can help your supervisees work through challenges that affect their attendance or performance. In particular, employees do not always know or understand FMLA protections, therefore, legally, you are required to tell them about FMLA, even if they do not directly ask for it. Had my supervisor worked with me and provided me options, I likely would have stayed in the job that I loved. And finally, a message to everyone, please remember to *"be kind, for everyone you meet is fighting a battle you know nothing about"* (Ian Maclaren, 1897).

Brooke (Boushon) Anderson, DNP, RN.

LinkedIn: www.linkedin.com/in/brookeanderson-dnp-rn

Just Two Dentists and a Hatred for Dentistry: *A Modern American Success Story?*

36

Joe Vaughn

I remember feeling relieved.

I sat on the floor of my bare empty apartment, my head resting against the back wall of my living room. Dirt and smudge and sweat speckled across my t-shirt. The last box had been loaded into the truck.

This was really happening.

As my wife and I sat there in our empty home, silent for what felt like hours, a million thoughts ran through our heads and through our hearts. Are we making the right decision? Is this worth it? What if we fail? Would it be too late to turn back?

Our somber gaze was met at eye level by the Space Needle staring back at us from a distance, the sun setting over the Olympic Mountains behind it. It was a sight whose beauty I had looked forward to every evening. But today was different. Today, the sunset meant that nothing would ever be the same again.

I had arrived in Seattle 6 years earlier almost to the day. A fresh bright-eyed graduate from dental school. Born and raised in Alabama, I wanted to use my 1-year residency as a chance to see a new part of the world, and it landed me in beautiful Seattle, WA. I fell in love with the city and the mountains, and then I fell in love with a girl, and "the rest was history," as they say.

But of course, the rest *wasn't* history.

I wish I could say that I had found my calling from the very beginning. I wish I could say that becoming a dentist was everything that everyone said it was going to be. I wish I could say that every day with a drill in my hand was my new favorite day. That I paid off my mountain of student debt with incredible ease. That every time I heard, *"Don't take this personally, but I really hate dentists,"* I, in fact, did not take it personally.

Oh, how I wish this was true. Things would have been a lot easier, that's for sure.

J. Vaughn (✉)
Department of Endodontics, Virginia Commonwealth University School of Dentistry, Richmond, VA, USA

But, of course, that's not how life tends to play out, is it? I'm assuming that if you're reading this right now, you may have an idea of where I'm coming from, whether you're a dentist or a physician or any one of the many healthcare professionals that dedicate their life to caring for others. Because the reality that we already know to be true is that our professions are extremely demanding. They're stressful. Emotionally draining. Not for the faint of heart. But what represents the much more troubling reality today is that we aren't supposed to talk about that part. We're supposed to be tough. Be professional. Leave your emotions at the door. *Never* show your cards. That, of course, precipitates into more stress, more anxiety, which ultimately becomes a yellow brick road to a potential career ending tragedy that we call "burnout."

So, is that just the way it is these days?

Not by a long shot.

I think that in our world today, it is *so* important that we challenge that story. Because the path to a rewarding, healthy career is lined with openness and honesty about those ups and those downs. We *need* to talk about them. Bring them to life. Because despite what you may see every day on Instagram, the real truth of our profession is that none of our careers is a healthy, happy, upward straight line. It's a wave. A series of them. We go up, we go down, we're all over the place.

Ask me how I know.

My wife and I have both struggled with burnout since we graduated dental school. "Purpose" was never a word we thought worthy of the work that we left our home every morning to go to. The past 6 years since graduation had been a perpetual search for wellness in our professional lives. Sure, there were some good times here and there. We loved the people we worked with. At times, we even *enjoyed* dentistry. But those waves were typically short-lived, and the reality set in that the dentistry we were a part of at the time made both of us feel incredibly unhappy and dissatisfied.

Being the analyzer I am, I tried countless times to pinpoint the reason. Why am I not happy being a general dentist? Aren't I lucky to be here? This wasn't supposed to happen, after all. I had been fed stories my entire life about how great it was to be a doctor. How I could have a meaningful purpose in life and even make a good living at the same time. How if I just worked hard in school, everything would take care of itself.

"Work hard now, and you'll be able to play for the rest of your life," my dad would always say, trying to convince me that studying was far more important than going out with my friends. This mentality continued all the way through dental school. Dentistry was that rewarding, respected "golf-every-Friday" career that everyone wanted to be a part of. I still remember while sitting in a practice management course, being encouraged by a corporate banker to take out as much student debt as we needed because dental practices *"never went under,"* and all of our financial worries would go away as soon as we landed our first job.

"Ah... that's the problem," I later realized.

The problem, at least in part, appears to be the alarming disconnect between the preconceived expectations of our professions and the true realities we experience in our first few years as a healthcare professional. No one really prepares you for the bad parts. No one tells you about the retired anesthesiologist that will someday look you dead in the eye and affirm that *"you may be a technician, but you're no real doctor."* No one tells you that 7 years out from graduation, you're still spending half of your paycheck on your student loans with literally decades left to go. No one tells you about how your profession isn't nearly as respected as you thought it was and that a *"thank you"* is sometimes few and far between.

Turns out, dentistry is *not* the solution to all my problems. It's not a golden ticket to success. For many, it hasn't been the guaranteed return on investment and it certainly hasn't been a career that automatically rewards you with joy, contentment and purpose just because you put in the effort.

So, if you think you're alone, you're wrong. You are *not* alone. And that's the first step to digging yourself out of a burnout situation. I was lucky in the fact that I knew I wasn't alone because my wife was a dentist and was just as unhappy as I was, even though we worked in totally separate work environments.

I don't think everyone is that lucky.

When I was a 3rd-year dental student serving on a national committee, the national President of American Student Dental Association took her own life in the middle of her final year of dental school. The news came as a terrible, heart wrenching shock. It hurts even now to think about how things might have been different if she had an outlet. It hurts to think about how things might have been different if we were more open and honest in our professions about the struggles our peers are likely facing every day.

We have to be better.

We have to be the voice that our professions really need. Let's talk about the things that no one thinks are okay to talk about. If you're out there suffering right now and no one knows it, you need to change that.

There *is* some good news in all of this, and it's that you can beat it. You can overcome the stress and anxiety and burnout. There's a never-ending list of resources out there, but ultimately you have to first recognize that you're struggling, and then you have to take action.

My wife and I were no different.

The thought struck us one day that we were basically just **two dentists who hated doing dentistry.**

For some reason, I never remember hearing *that* particular American success story when I was younger. But something tells me that we aren't the only ones. Six years spent searching for our place in the profession. Six years desperately hoping we would find something somewhere that could bring us joy in our work lives, only to have it lead us to packing our whole life up in a truck and moving 3000 miles away.

It wasn't easy. Many conversations, many arguments, and a few sets of tears went into our decision. But ultimately, we both decided to leave our jobs as general dentists. I made a tough decision to go back to school and was lucky enough to get accepted into endodontic residency in Richmond, VA. My wife was coming with me with no job and absolutely no social connections in our new home state.

If a profession truly is a series of waves, then that day sitting on the floor of our empty Seattle apartment was certainly a melancholic trough.

But of course, it didn't last, just like it never really does.

It's been 18 months since that day in our Seattle apartment, and things feel a bit different now. I'm back in school, a resident once more. Literally thousands of miles away from my general dentistry days, but it's the very first time in my career that I've felt content in an operatory. Felt like everything is in its right place. For the very first time, I have a glimpse of that elusive sense of purpose that I've heard so much about.

And my wife? She's now a full-time faculty member at the dental school. When we first moved to Virginia, she took 4 months off from working. As it turns out, that brief 'sabbatical' alone did wonders for her emotional wellness and ultimately helped her refocus and define what she wanted from her career.

That led to what has turned out to be the best job she has ever had, the start of what will likely be a lifelong career in academia. The work she's doing these days is finally "purpose" worthy, and I can attest that I have never seen her happier.

Will this last? Is *this* the "and-the-rest-was-history" ending that we've been looking for?

I don't know, really.

Something tells me that life probably has a few more waves in store for us. But to be honest with you, the waves aren't as scary anymore. I'm not worried for the future like I was some years back. And it's because of these experiences that we've shared. Because of these terrible lows and amazing highs. Because of that silent evening on our empty apartment floor. That willingness to pivot. To leave our careers and our lives behind and travel 3000 miles in search of a metaphorical land of milk and honey.

I've thought an awful lot about dentistry over the first few years of my career. The ups and the downs. Healthcare has the potential to be the most rewarding career on the planet. But it can just as easily cause enormous detriment to someone's life. So much so that it can make you feel completely powerless, like you have no one to talk to and nowhere to go.

Everyone has a place in this profession. But not everyone finds it at the same time or stage in their career.

So, if you aren't happy with where you are right now, keep searching for your right place. The worst thing that I can imagine in this world is to spend your entire career dreading the commute to work every morning. Be willing to make the pivot when necessary. Sure, it may be scary. You'll have many questions, and they may not all get answered. You may even find yourself sitting on the floor of an empty apartment trying to imagine what life will look like in 6 months.

I've been there.

But what I've learned is that on the other side of that moment... on the other side of that decision to pivot... it's not quite as scary as it may first appear.

Joe Vaughn, DMD

He/him

@jvaughn_dmd

Taking the Wheel

37

Tracy Asamoah

"I think I want to be a doctor when I grow up," 12-year-old me casually mentioned to my parents one day after school. I liked science, but I liked art and writing too. My statement was more of a musing than a declaration. But, in speaking those words, I opened the door to a cacophony of voices that would attempt to direct my life choices.

Once my parents got a notion of my interest, my future was decided. It wasn't that a college or even advanced degree was a new accomplishment for my family. I'm not the first person or even part of the first generation in my family to go to college. My parents grew up two black kids in the Jim Crow south. In a time of turmoil and violence, their parents saw education as a ticket to freedom and opportunity. My parents, both receiving their master's degrees, wanted no less for me than their parents wanted for them. Their daughter had an interest in and the skills for becoming a doctor. They were going to make sure that it happened.

Once I put my idea out into the world, it took on a life of its own. The small voice, barely above a whisper, that wondered *"what if?"* was soon overshadowed by a loving and well-intentioned but insistent chorus of family and friends. They weren't going to be deterred from sending the family's first future doctor to medical school. Without them, I'm certain that I wouldn't have made it all the way through. Their support buoyed me as I explored and flailed in unfamiliar territories. However, along the way, their voices drowned out my own.

Having inherited a strong internal drive and perseverance from my dad, I pushed through my education and training. I didn't question my goal. I didn't even ask myself what my goal really was. A medical degree waited on the horizon. As a kid, whenever anyone asked me why I wanted to be a doctor, my responses felt generic.

"I want to take care of people."

"I like science."

Yet the answers to basic, deeper questions perplexed me.

T. Asamoah (✉)
Washington, DC, USA

"How will you know when you've been successful?"
"When will enough be enough?"

I knew why my mom wanted me to be a doctor, what my dad measured as success and what my 3rd year med school surgery attending thought was enough (nothing, ever). So, I listened to these voices and pressed on, checking the boxes, but often feeling like I was falling short. As a healthy, young person working her way down the medical training pathway, this worked for a while.

I completed medical school, residency, and fellowship and began the life of an attending physician at a nearby medical school. I was taking care of patients, exploring research, and teaching students and trainees. Three more boxes checked. However, I had never felt more lost and confused about what I was doing.

During this first year as a junior faculty member, it all changed. One morning in the shower, I noticed tingling in my left hand. It had the pins and needles sensation I'd experienced from many poorly positioned naps. The "waking up" continued for several days. There were other things too. I was a bit more tired than usual. However, as a fresh out of fellowship junior faculty member, I considered that part of the job. Strange, new sensations down my back were a different story. If I moved my head in just the right (or wrong) way, a tiny lightning bolt shot down my spine.

For a while, I dismissed it. Our new German Shepard puppy, Malachi, had been dragging me through his daily walks. Maybe it was just run of the mill tendonitis from our rambunctious pup. Eventually, I had to acknowledge that the tingling sensation in my hand and shocks down my back weren't normal. My hand felt like a block of ice that was slowly melting, and ignoring it wasn't helping me.

For the first time in my life, my body was forcing me to listen to a different voice. This internal voice was telling me that something was off in my body that couldn't be ignored. Not quite ready to head this voice's warning, I consulted my husband. He had just started his ER residency training. His brain was all rapid diagnosis and treatment planning. After several days of waiting for my hand to thaw, I mentioned my symptoms to him.

"Sounds like MS to me." No physical exam or further questioning. Just the first diagnosis that came to his mind that best explained the symptoms I had described. He wasn't wrong. I had considered the possibility that I might have a legitimate neurological issue. However, at 30 years old, newly married and hoping to start a family soon, I wasn't ready to hear that I might have a chronic, potentially life altering, illness. Nowhere in my parents' advice was guidance about what to do if my career got derailed. Multiple Sclerosis wasn't on the path that I had meticulously followed since I was 12 years old. My body was now calling the shots and I realized that I was going to have to turn my attention inward and start listening to, and trusting, my own voice.

Life has gifted me important lessons since my initial diagnosis. Not in one revelatory moment, but in a slow process of surrender, self-reflection, and acceptance. This process has allowed for growth and discovery that might not have been available to me had I not been forced to focus on my physical health.

First, I learned that I can only truly be whom I'm meant to be in the world when I stop leading with the external voices. Expectations from those closest to me as well as the larger society have impact and meaning in my life. These external voices have inspired, motivated, and pushed me towards the various goals I've set for myself. However, these external expectations are secondary to the expectations I have for myself. Those external voices are both the invited and uninvited passengers in my car on the road of my life journey, but I'm behind the wheel. They have all sorts of thoughts and opinions about where we should go and how we should get there. Ultimately, only I can truly visualize the destination that's best for me and design a path forward. I can choose to accept or reject their input and trust that either way, I'm fully capable of living with the consequences of my choices.

I've also realized that even though I'm a physician, my identity is not wholly wrapped up in this title. My medical training was a beginning, not the destination. Becoming a physician has been an important component of who I am, but it has only been a single point in the arc of my life story. My diagnosis opened the door for me to consider options for using my skillset as a physician in ways other than practicing clinical medicine. My inner voice reminds me to explore options that allow me to design a career that promotes wellness and is sensitive to my limitations.

Finally, I'm paying attention to an important voice that I long ignored. My body. My body holds wisdom, so now I include it in my life planning. Managing my auto-immune disorder means prioritizing those things that help slow its progression. My focus centers on flourishing, not disease. This means getting adequate quality sleep, eating a plant-focused diet, and staying physically active. When I don't do these things, my body sends my brain warning signals. One poor night's sleep guarantees that I'll be less focused and more irritable the next day.

All of this has allowed me to envision who I truly want to be as a physician. I'm guided by what I know to be true about and right for me. However, I can also welcome and hold the opinions of all those other passengers in the car. When they get too loud and try to take the wheel, I just turn up the music and keep on driving.

Tracy Asamoah, MD, ACC
Outpatient Child and Adolescent Psychiatry
Career and Transition Coach
https://www.tracyasamoahmd.com/
https://www.tracyasamoahcoaching.com/

When Life Hands You Lemons

Sarah Wilczewski

It's no secret—the mental health crisis is real. We hear about it every day in the news, through social media, and even on billboards. Despite these constant reminders, it's hard to truly grasp the extent and severity of this problem until you've been there yourself. That's what led me here today.

As a seasoned health care professional, I felt like I was mentally and physically prepared for anything. After graduating from the University of Wisconsin School of Nursing, I spent 2 years working as a Registered Nurse in both the Neurosciences and Trauma Intensive Care Units. Patients in these ICUs are the sickest of the sick—oftentimes clinging to life on ventilators and multiple vasoactive medication infusions. The work was stressful, both physically and emotionally, but nothing I couldn't handle. To be honest, I thrived in this environment.

After an additional few years of demanding anesthesia training, I obtained my Masters in Nurse Anesthesia from the Mayo Clinic College of Medicine. For the next 10 years, I would spend my days providing anesthesia care for patients undergoing a variety of surgical procedures, from the completely healthy college athlete to the critically ill trauma patient. Emergencies would arise on occasion, and I would respond appropriately and efficiently—that is our job as anesthesia providers. We are there to ensure that patients wake up quickly, safely, and pain-free, regardless of any unexpected intraoperative events.

One morning, all of this would change. Shortly after making the surgical incision for an elective procedure, my otherwise healthy patient went into cardiac arrest. After providing resuscitative measures for nearly an hour, it was determined that our efforts were futile. My patient never made it off the operating room table that day. Throughout the resuscitation, I remained calm, focused, and determined. As soon as the time of death was pronounced, I completely fell apart. It is our duty as anesthetists to fix any problem that arises, no matter how big or small—but I couldn't fix this.

S. Wilczewski (✉)
Revival Infusion Madison, Fitchburg, WI, USA
e-mail: info@revivalinfusion.com

In the following days I replayed the scenes of that day constantly through my mind. My thoughts were all over the place. I felt sadness, guilt, anger, uncertainty, and overwhelming anxiety. I woke up with an elephant on my chest every morning and couldn't close my eyes without reliving those few hours. I questioned everything—why this patient? Why was I assigned to that case? Why am I struggling, while everyone else seems to be doing just fine? I knew that mine was the last face my patient saw, and the last voice they heard. Did I say the right thing? Did I make that person feel safe and comfortable?

I spent the next several weeks in this state of debilitating anxiety. I couldn't sleep, felt constantly on edge and experienced daily panic attacks. I cried over seemingly nothing and felt myself growing short with my husband and two young sons. I couldn't work—I could barely get through the motions of the day. While navigating these symptoms, I reached out to dozens of therapy and psychiatry groups in the area, only to be told that nearly all providers had a 3–6-month waitlist (if they were accepting new patients at all). This led to further exhaustion and feelings of discouragement.

Once I was able to connect with a therapist, I was officially diagnosed with PTSD and began months of intense therapy. My therapist recommended EMDR (Eye Movement Desensitization and Reprocessing) therapy, which is a form of therapy especially effective for the treatment of PTSD. I was fortunate in that I responded extremely well to EMDR. Therapy was intense and emotionally draining, but with each session I could feel my symptoms slowly improving. However, as the old saying goes, *"when it rains, it pours"*. During this time, I received word that a close family member of my husband had taken her life as a result of postpartum depression. It was in that moment, at my lowest of lows, that I was inspired to make a change.

Mental illness is something that has always been close to my mind and heart. In my first semester of Nursing School, my 12-year-old cousin committed suicide. My mother-in-law battled alcoholism as long as I knew her. Now, having recently lost another family member to suicide and personally experiencing PTSD, I felt the push to shift gears professionally.

I knew there had to be a way to use my training and skills as an anesthesia provider to make a difference in the mental health arena. It didn't take long to land on the answer: ketamine. While ketamine itself is an anesthesia medication, it has proven its value as a powerful tool in the treatment of depression and other mood disorders. I enrolled in an online course, the Ketamine Academy, geared towards teaching medical professionals the ins and outs of owning and operating a successful clinic. I met with a team of healthcare attorneys, read dozens of research articles, and dove headfirst into opening my own practice. Within a few short months, I officially resigned from the hospital and opened Revival Infusion Madison—the very first dedicated ketamine infusion clinic in the Madison area.

Since February of 2022, I have been treating patients with a variety of mental health disorders, including treatment-resistant depression, PTSD, anxiety, severe postpartum depression, and suicidal ideation. I have witnessed severely depressed patients—including patients who have made multiple suicide attempts in the past year—turn their lives around. Many of these are people you would never suspect of silently suffering: accomplished physicians, thriving business owners, college athletes, dentists, therapists, and nurses, just to name a few. I've laughed and cried with patients, heard stories you wouldn't believe, and been the recipient of the most heartfelt hugs. It has been the most fulfilling role of my career.

If someone had told me a year ago what I'd be doing today, I never would have believed it. I know it sounds cheesy, but I've always been a believer in the sentiment, *"everything happens for a reason"*. I think back to the days immediately following that OR case often. I no longer question the reasoning behind my involvement that day, because I now see the bigger picture. It still makes me sad that a patient lost their life in my presence—but I truly believe I've saved countless other lives as a result. It's helped me become a more present and patient mother and wife, and a more compassionate provider.

All in all, I've learned a lot of lessons this past year. Mental health is vitally important. Too many people suffer in silence, wearing a mask to get through their days. Nobody is immune from mental illness, no matter how tough you think you are. Identify your support systems and lean on them in times of need. Kindness and compassion matter. There's often a silver lining, even when it's hard to identify. If you see an opportunity, take it. When life hands you lemons, make lemonade. And lastly, but most importantly, never give up on yourself.

Sarah Wilczewski, CRNA, APNP

https://www.revivalinfusion.com/

Healing from Burnout Through Reinvention: A Change Will Do You Good

39

Rosalind Kaplan

The first time I thought about leaving medicine came early in my career. As an internist who did primary care in the office and also rounded in the hospital, full weekends off were rare, and weekdays were long. I was in my 30's, had two children under 10 years old and a husband, also an internist, who had big ambitions in academic medicine. I bounced from one academic hospital system to another, and finally landed with three other female internists in a brand-new, hospital-owned community practice.

The practice was popular and successful from the beginning; our patient panels grew quickly. Too quickly. Within 3 years of opening the practice, our schedules were entirely full. I had a following of patients with complex medical and psychosocial needs. The administration believed in overbooking our 15-min appointments, so it was just about guaranteed we'd run late, and my particular clientele often needed some extra time and TLC, which further crunched my time. I hustled about, seeing patients, returning calls, running back and forth to the hospital for admissions and rounds before and after patient hours. I stopped having time for lunch. Then I stopped having time for bathroom breaks, and soon I was also staying late in the evenings to review labs and write my notes in oaktag charts filled with lined paper.

When I left the office, I'd rush to collect my kids from school and day care, praying I wouldn't be the last parent to make it to pick up. The evening progressed with dinner, baths, and bedtime, and I'd fall into bed, exhausted, ready to do it over in the morning, or sooner, if I was on call and my pager woke me during the night.

For those of us who did rigorous residencies with overnight call every third night, this sort of lifestyle felt 'normal.' But in reality, I was chronically exhausted, and my health suffered on every level. I had only 6 weeks off for maternity leave for each child, unpaid. This was not enough time to recover physically and get a baby on a regular schedule, much less to fend off a postpartum depression. When my mother

R. Kaplan (✉)
Sidney Kimmel Medical College, Philadelphia, PA, USA

died suddenly at the age of 62, I was expected to turn around and get back to work a week later. When a medical issue landed me on toxic medications for a year, I pushed through my side effects and showed up for rounds and office hours without missing a beat. *'Pull yourself up by the bootstraps'* was the name of the game, and I played it, over and over again, until those bootstraps wore out and snapped.

A decade into my life as an attending physician, I considered leaving the profession. Friends outside of medicine seemed happier, more balanced, more financially secure, and certainly better-rested than I did. I was worried that my kids were spending too much time at school or with babysitters. But I truly loved my patients and the challenge of taking good care of them. I got a lot of positive reinforcement for my 'bedside manner', and for my skill at diagnosis and treatment. Besides, what else did I know how to do?

I wasn't ready for a whole new career. But I did need a change. I spoke to experts in practice management, friends in private practice, a private business consultant.

"You have the kind of patients who require extra time. You should bill for your time, like a psychiatrist," one consultant told me.

"Insurance doesn't pay enough for this kind of patient to get what they need," said another. *"You should try a fee-for-service model, in which patients pay the office directly and then submit claims,"* said another.

Today, we'd call this 'Direct Care.' 'Concierge' medicine would also have allowed me to give patients extra time and care without suffering financially, but in the 1990s, these were not tried and true practice models. Still, I was ready to try it. I opened a solo, out-of-network office, and did things my way. A good management consultant made up for my lack of business acumen and skills, and soon one of my partners from my previous practice decided to join me. We made it work for 13 years. We didn't make a lot of money, but we did medicine the way we were taught to do it- with our full attention, a lot of heart, and adequate time for each patient.

I was happy in this situation. Working for myself, I could plan my time so I didn't miss my kids' sports events or need to scramble if a child was sick. In this model, I even had some energy left over for creative pursuits. For me, it was writing. Narrative medicine, some family memoir, some personal essays. I'd never been a writer in college, and had taken few writing classes, but I was a voracious reader. I taught myself, and also attended writing workshops for more help. Writing helped me process the hard things: my patient's struggles, my mother's sudden death, the challenges of parenting and family life.

It would have been nice to continue that pace for a few more years. But time moves forward, the world changes, kids grow, and technology pushes ahead. 2008 brought a recession, and we lost patients who found themselves struggling financially; it was too expensive to have medical insurance and also put money up front for visits. Soon after, Medicare mandates for EMRs pulled us, kicking and screaming, into the digital world. The expenses and pressures of technology were too much for our low-profile practice.

My kids left for college right around the same time. Without carpools, after school sports, and curriculum nights, I could throw myself into work more fully. I was offered a position in an academic general medical section. My clinical work would be primary care of women, and I'd also be helping to develop a multidisciplinary women's center. I was excited—I could envision an ideal environment for women's health, with primary care, mental health, gyn, nutrition, breast care and osteoporosis management all under one roof, and as medical school faculty, I'd be teaching medical students and residents again.

Maybe the dive was too deep, in retrospect. I'd already been taking care of everyone but myself for more than two decades. I was good at taking care of others, and I took it seriously. My patient practice grew quickly again, and I took my students and trainees under my wing. I also saw the women's clinic as 'my baby', but, unlike my other children, it didn't thrive. Academic politics and institutional finances kept putting roadblocks in the way. The women's clinic never came to fruition, and the multidisciplinary care of my complicated patients continued to fall to me alone; the institutional and practice support were both inadequate and dysfunctional. My patient schedule was always full and my inbox overflowed each day. I was back to having no time for lunch or bathroom breaks. Now, in the digital era, I stayed late, but I also brought hours of work home each night.

Six years into this, I wasn't just tired or a little frazzled. I was fried. Feeling depressed, demoralized, and utterly alone, I began to think it might time to hang up my stethoscope for good. I truly felt broken at that point—I cried on the way to work and on the way home, and I was often too tired to do much outside of work. I tried to do 'self-care.' I went to therapy, I tried to exercise, I took a yoga and meditation class. It didn't make a dent.

Writing had remained a solace and a tool during all of these years. I wrote stories and essays, attended a writing workshop one evening a week, and taught narrative medicine workshops and classes off and on. I always felt like I had to really squeeze the writing in; I never really had the time. When my husband or my therapist asked me what I wanted to do if I didn't want to practice medicine, I said I wanted to write. And not necessarily about medicine. Medicine had sucked up all my energy for 30 years. I wanted myself back.

While I contemplated leaving my job, I started researching writing programs. Not sure if I was serious, I applied to a few, sending work that I'd polished in my weekly workshop. A few months later, I was accepted into a low-residency MFA program with a generous scholarship attached. I knew I couldn't keep my job and also earn my MFA. Some people do, but they have 9–5 jobs that they leave in the office. I decided to take another dive.

The day I walked out of my academic office for the last time, I was outwardly composed. I'd stopped crying after I resigned from my faculty position. I'd put my mind to wrapping up my business there, assuring that my patients had follow-up care and saying goodbye to students and colleagues. It was hard to explain my plan to study writing, which seemed like such a non-sequitur. Worse, I worried it sounded useless, as once it had to me, when I'd seen 'value' only in what I did for others. But I would soon find out that when we do more for ourselves, we have more to give to others.

Two years later, in 2020, I got my MFA. Graduation was online, our degrees conferred over Zoom during the pre-vaccine part of the pandemic. I also, by then, had a stable part-time job with an urgent care company, seeing patients and supervising physician assistants. The MFA was exactly what I needed—concerted time to let my left brain heal while my right brain came back alive, and to figure out what came next. As I healed, I began to miss medicine, to crave the puzzle pieces of diagnosis, the satisfaction of successful treatment and even the challenge of uncertainty. Urgent Care, in its specifics, was an accident, but it also made sense. My emotional being was satisfied by writing and teaching; I could still help patients, still use my medical brain, still earn a living, and still have my days off free to write and to take care of myself. I soon added a day weekly in a clinic for uninsured patients as a volunteer primary care physician.

The icing on the cake is that I now teach writing for medical students again, and I do it with a little twist. Instead of asking them to write patient narratives, I ask them to write about themselves. Patient care retains a role in their writing, but instead of using writing specifically to bear witness to the patient, with the goal of better patient care, they write about their own stories, their feelings, their needs, who they were and are and hope to be. Healing for them, this writing is a kind of self-care, a tool they can take with them for the rest of their lives. Within a class, writing binds them to each other, teaching empathy for each other and for self. Paradoxically, this does exactly what it didn't set out to do. It makes them better doctors because it allows them to be human.

I'm near the natural end of my career now. Near, but not at, not yet. This cocktail of a career is working for me right now. I've learned to anticipate the next step, plan for the next transition. For me, that will be coaching other physicians to make their careers work for them, something I can do indefinitely, even if my aging body is no longer up to fast-paced clinical care. I'm starting a coaching certification course this fall. Stay tuned.

Rosalind Kaplan, MD, FACP, MFA
she/her/hers
Associate Professor of Clinical Medicine, Adjunct
Sidney Kimmel Medical College, Philadelphia, PA
drrozkaplan.com

From Stillbirth to Mindfulness and Community

Amy Pelkey

One diagnostic test changed our lives forever as the ultrasound tech uttered the words, *"I can't find a heartbeat."* We knew going into the exam that our daughter, Anna Grace, was sick. But no amount of knowledge fully prepares you to lose a baby.

Two weeks prior, a severe cystic hygroma and ascites had been detected during a routine prenatal ultrasound. A full work-up began. Genetic tests did not reveal any abnormalities. A congenital heart condition was not detected. We were told Anna had life limiting conditions, without a clear cause. After carefully weighing our options, we continued the pregnancy and focused on palliative care options until she passed inside of me.

On September 23, 2016, after being induced, we cherished our day with Anna. Her blue eyes and distinct chin shape reminded us of our son. We took pictures, held a heartfelt service for her, and cried a lot. I vividly remember holding her hand between my thumb and index finger, cradling her body, and then saying our final good-byes. Leaving our daughter behind, as we walked out of the hospital, was heartbreaking.

At the time, both my husband and I worked as CRNAs at an academic, Level 1 trauma center where Anna was born. Some of our colleagues had become our care givers adding another layer of support to an already strong network of family and friends.

Despite this support, going to therapy, and taking a full maternity leave, I felt lonely. I spent countless hours searching online and in bereavement groups on Facebook, hoping to connect with other grieving healthcare providers. I longed to hear their stories and learn how they navigated the challenges of returing to clinical practice while surrounded by triggers.

A. Pelkey, (✉)
Pause to Remember, Washington, PA, USA
e-mail: amy@pausetoremember.org; amy@amypelkey.com

Over the course of the first year, two coping patterns emerged. On maternity leave, I numbed my pain with reality TV, junk food, and wine. As I returned to work, I found myself setting new goals to challenge and distract myself to the point of exhaustion. Thankfully, these maladaptive choices were occasionally interrupted by books, such as *Man's Search for Meaning* by Viktor Frankl, and the mindfulness practices I had learned in a course called Mindfulness Based Stress Reduction (MBSR).

Developed by Jon Kabat-Zinn in 1979, MBSR encompasses various mindfulness practices such as meditation, yoga, mindful eating and walking. Mindfulness provided me a Sanctuary to process my emotions without judgement. It allowed me freedom from the chaos in my mind and numbness or tension in my body. Each time I stepped onto my mat or sat in meditation, peace and solace followed. It felt like a break from my grief.

To deepen my yoga practice, I enrolled in a 200-hour yoga teacher training (YTT), program through a local yoga studio, four months after Anna's passing. Over seven months, my tear-filled yoga mat, broken heart, and sporadic attempts to teach yoga were met with warmth, encouragement, and the gift of friendship from the other trainees.

During YTT, I met another grief mother who had experienced multiple losses and had one living daughter. Together we founded Pause to Remember in the fall of 2017. We offered a two-hour grief-based meditation and yoga workshop held in various yoga studios in the Greater Pittsburgh area. Unfortunately, our limited marketing plan resulted in fewer participants than we had hoped for. Nevertheless, I knew we were onto something at the conclusion of one workshop when a grieving mother shared that she experienced relief from a persistent headache for the first time in weeks.

My incessant goal setting left little time for Pause To Remember after the first year. Instead, I accepted a position on the Lead CRNA team and said "yes" to committee work. Our work schedules evolved to include beeper and then in-house night call. Break and lunch coverage was thinning. The mounting clinical stressors took a toll on me while I continued to work through my grief. Within two years, I dropped my hours in the hospital to work in a ketamine clinic hoping the change would calm my burnout. It only intensified it.

At this I point, I needed help and sought guidance from burnout coach, Dr. Errin Weisman. Working with her felt like hitting a reset button as I realigned my priorities. Self-care, family, teaching yoga, and Pause to Remember were again at the top of my list.

My work with Dr. Weisman carried me until the pandemic hit. COVID-19 closed the two yoga studios where I taught. I found myself navigating virtual learning with our second grade son amidst the uncertainty and stress in the hospital. Despite these challenges, I decided this was the time to revamp Pause to Remember to an online offering. I did not know where to start. My friend and co-founder had moved into the yoga for cancer space. She gave permission to take over Pause to Remember independently. Having no tech skills, I enrolled in some online courses. Building websites, email automations, and trying yoga on Zoom turned out to be time consuming, challenging, and more rewarding than I anticipated.

Evan after constructing the website, writing an eBook, and designing a course, I struggled to build the online community. Seeking guidance, I turned to Krista Kehoe, a life coach specializing in women with online offerings and businesses. With her assistance, I identified the burnout fueled by the pandemic, the stress of staffing shortages, and weight of pregnancy and infant loss among female, licensed healthcare providers. These insights reshaped Pause to Remember into what it is today: a community dedicated to supporting healthcare providers grieving after a miscarriage, ectopic pregnancy, c-section with hysterectomy, termination for medical reasons, stillbirth, or infant loss.

The offerings are evolving. Currently, a monthly virtual support group, Facebook group, virtual yoga pop-up classes, and eBook are offered freely. The Pause to Remember Podcast features resources, meditations, and healthcare providers sharing their loss and grief journeys while preserving the memory of their baby (or babies). The goal is to normalize difficult conversations and let others know they are not alone.

In addition, an online 4-week, mindfulness-based grief support course specifically tailored for grieving healthcare providers, called MNDFL Rx (Mindful Prescription), has been created. This course incorporates meditation, yoga, and other informal mindfulness practices to help providers build courage to acknowledge and process their feelings, strength to carry the weight of their grief, and resilience so they can find a new norm after loss. MNDFL Rx will be offered online in a group format and as a private, one-to-one option beginning January 2023.

There is evidence suggesting that pregnancy and infant loss is more common in healthcare providers. For instance, research published in *JAMA Surgery,* in 2021 revealed 42% of female surgeons had experienced pregnancy loss compared to about 20–25% in the general population (Rangel et al. 2021). Only other providers who have endured this type of loss can have an appreciation for the aftermath that follows.

For the past six years, my journey has been transformative. Shifting to a per diem schedule allowed me to homeschool our son since the start of the pandemic, teach yoga, and support the Pause to Remember community. It feels rewarding to redirect my care from hospital patients to grieving providers who are navigating through one of the darkest periods of their lives. Sometimes simply holding space and being present is enough.

Yoga has taught me that everything changes and everything ends. Mindfulness has helped me release labels like "good" or "bad." Although the story I mentally wrote for Anna when the pregnancy test turned positive took an unexpected turn, I have chosen not to label Anna's passing as "bad." Instead, the untainted ripples of her brief life flow unobstructed through Pause to Remember. She is my beacon and our precious gift.

To every provider grieving after pregnancy or infant loss, please know you have the power to slow down, establish boundaries, and tend to your own physical, mental, and emotional needs. Pregnancy and infant loss reshapes life in profound ways, often making time feel suspended. However, grieving providers can choose how they want to navigate their grief, find others to support them through a heart-breaking journey, and discover unique ways to honor their baby's life.

The one universal truth about grief is that it is a unique journey without a predetermined timeframe. There is no right or wrong path to follow-only your own grieving path. Mapping the passage through grief includes unanticipated stops, U-turns, and moments of feeling lost. Yet there are tools available that serve as a compass and provide support along the way. In the Pause to Remember community, there is space for any female healthcare provider grieving the loss of their baby. You will be welcomed with open arms and your baby's precious memory will be honored.

Amy Pelkey, MSN, CRNA, RYT 200

(she/her)

Founder of Pause to Remember, CRNA, Yoga Teacher

https://www.pausetoremember.org/

Podcast: Pause to Remember

IG/FB: @pausetoremember

Email: amy@pausetoremember.org

Reference

Rangel EL, Castillo-Angles M, Easter SR, et al. Incidence of infertility and pregnancy complications in US female surgeons. JAMA Surg. 2021;156(10):905–15. https://doi.org/10.1001/JAMAsurg.2021.3301.

How to Fine Tune Mental Health: The Power of Social Prescription

41

Anita Bangale

A few years ago, I took care of a 16-year-old male named Jordan. He has no idea how profoundly he changed my life. Like many young patients, Jordan had no significant past medical history, but his mother had convinced him to check in to the emergency department out of concern for his worsening mental health. He ended up getting diagnosed with severe depression, requiring inpatient treatment. By the time I saw him, he had been waiting days simply to get admitted to a psychiatry unit. The main issue—there were no beds available in the entire city, so he ended up being held in limbo in the emergency department for more than a week to get the care he desperately needed. On one of those days, he stopped me while I was briskly walking down to the hall to assess a critical patient. Honestly, I was annoyed. I didn't have time for another interruption. *"Doc,"* he said, with the most earnest look in his eyes, *"I feel helpless."* I paused and looked back, surprised by his courage and vulnerability. I wanted to say something more hopeful, but replied truthfully, *"so do I."*

I knew Jordan's extraordinary wait for specialized care was not any one person's fault, and there was very little in my control. So, what could I do? I chose to be bold. I broke hospital policy and let him do something that was not permitted. I let him play his choice of music in the hallways of the emergency department while waiting for the psychiatric unit to open up a bed. With that seemingly simple act, the effect on Jordan, myself and our whole team during that shift was profound. We learned Jordan learned to play guitar and piano at the age of 8 and he proudly guided his band as the lead guitarist. For him, music created happiness. Through this simple act of letting him press play, we offered him a dose of therapy amidst chaos. This interaction made me realize how deeply I needed to press play on my own hobbies. Dance, reading and cooking were not passions that needed to pass in the wake of training, rather they were essential catalysts that I needed to pursue in order to continue succeeding as a physician.

A. Bangale (✉)
Bangale Emergency Solutions, Houston, TX, USA

In the ER and throughout medicine, we are exposed not just to the medically sick, but also to the deeper social issues facing our communities. We witness the most raw elements—poverty, drugs, abuse, and mental health issues. Our natural instinct may be to look away from the complex mental health component, but we know it's there in the ether. Over time, I have grown to open my eyes wide and even run towards the complex mental health issues. It's certainly not easy, but I see that mental health colors so much of the patient and provider experience. As I think about it more, our mental health is at the core of every human experience. After my interaction with Jordan, I couldn't help but wonder…maybe we all need a little music?

I have thought a lot about Jordan since that shift—specifically, how much he connected to the songs playing in the background. The music's impact went far beyond passing time until he got the right bed. It seemed to bring out a dormant happiness. Now, when I look around at my colleagues, I see so many who are yearning to find joy in medicine and in life again. And I think about my own passions and hobbies, and realize, they too nourish my soul and serve as a platform to connect with others—almost like an antidote to loneliness. I have thought more about how these connections to our interests are at the core of human fulfillment and learned about an entire practice in the UK, Australia and Canada called social prescription.

Social prescription is a treatment strategy that improves health and wellbeing through simple behaviors that link us to our passions kind of like a prescription pad for the arts or nature. Think about an activity you enjoy—maybe it's playing soccer or painting or meeting up with your book club. Imagine if someone else in healthcare literally prescribed these activities for you. For me, a weekly dose of dance class would naturally elevate my mood because of the dopamine hit from the movement itself, but also because of the connection with people who share the same passion. For someone working to lower their cholesterol level, their prescription might include a daily walk with a neighbor and a healthy cooking class. And for someone in medicine working to improve their sense of confidence and self-worth after a poor patient outcome, their prescription could suggest a peer group to recognize and self-monitor feelings.

In general, social prescription involves simple solutions like phone calls, walks, or volunteering. You might wonder, are we all not participating in these activities already? Unfortunately, no. It's the stuff many of us wish we did, but don't, especially in today's healthcare world filled with charting, paperwork and metrics. In such a busy and booked culture, we tend to fill the white spaces of our calendars with obligations that leave us drained. The simple pleasures of social prescription are the first to go because we deem them optional or even selfish. And our need for companionship is often ignored, especially as we feel surrounded by staff and patients all day. But I challenge that the elements of social prescription are the very basic requirements of healthy mental health, and even more critical for those of us in medicine to pursue this goal. The more we are aware and participate in our own personal social prescription, the better we will feel and the healthier and more energized we will actually become.

And THAT boost is something our medical community absolutely needs right now. Alarmingly, mental health challenges are the leading cause of disability and poor life outcomes in young people. Depression is at least as common in the medical profession as in the general population, affecting an estimated 12% of males and up to 19.5% of females. Depression is even more common in medical students and residents, with 15–30% of them screening positive for depressive symptoms. More than 4 in 10 adults in the US show symptoms of depression or anxiety, and we lose nearly one doctor a day to suicide (Goebert et al. 2009; Goldman et al. 2015; Khadilkar 2022; Schwenk 2015). Despite the numbers, many of us choose to ignore the topic altogether and dismiss mental health as an overplayed buzzword or as something affecting "those kinds of people." But those people are the very people we see daily, in our hallways and hospitals, and looking back at us in the mirror. It is high time we bridge the gap in knowledge and understanding—and equip ourselves with simple tools to restore healthy mental health in medicine. **Let's stop treating mental health—let's start integrating it.**

Each of us has the power to change the status quo and integrate social prescription into our own lives. Will it work? Let's look at the data. We know that loneliness and social isolation are major risk factors for mental illness, especially depression. A 2010 study from over 300,000 elderly individuals found that loneliness can present as great a mortality risk as smoking 15 cigarettes a day (Holt-Lunstad et al. 2010). Activities such as choir singing, art-making, expressive writing and group drumming reduce mental distress, and at the time, improve individual and social well-being.

The data also shows us that people tend to stick to the activities of social prescription because of how enjoyable they are. People feel connected socially, and we see a spike in oxytocin—our love hormone—and dopamine—our neurotransmitter of joy. And furthermore, behavioral activation takes place—which means the more regularly and consistently we do positive things for ourselves, the higher our self-esteem and independence.

So, think about your colleague who seems to be more withdrawn lately… suppose you invite them on a walk one day. This simple ask has the potential to improve their quality of life as you build a bridge of connection, eliminate loneliness, and improve independence. In fact, you may help them re-discover their own music.

But there's more we can do. What if we also used this tool of social prescription to support medical students and residents to help mitigate the rise of depression and anxiety in these groups? Medical schools and residency programs are environments that serve as the first line of defense for students and those in training. We know that depression can compromise our ability to form relationships and set goals. So, if we can teach this group how to manage mental health early on, this can impact and improve their entire personal and professional careers.

I propose that students and residents have access to a navigator, similar to an emotional coach—the same way they have access to extra time in the anatomy lab. The navigator is emotionally invested in each individual's success and has spent time and energy before and during the school year getting to know the student— their passions, motivations, and goals. Together with the navigator, the trainee has created an algorithm—designed specifically for them—anticipating stressors, based on their individual values and priorities. So, when they fail a test or have a poor patient outcome or get the wrong answer on rounds, each person already has an SOS plan in place. It's a proactive approach that responds, relatively early on, before any major conflict has developed. The navigator's objective is to ask the student "*What matters to you?*" instead of wondering "*What's the matter with you?*" They're aware that having depression and anxiety shouldn't be a big deal but having empowering and innovative solutions should be. I believe we can ultimately make a navigator role a reality in our medical schools and residency programs. However, what we can all do right now is serve as a navigator for ourselves and our colleagues.

It's time to reimagine a world in medicine where we take charge of our mental health simply. Let us create the sense of belonging we all crave so that like Jordan, we can all hear our own music, regardless of the world's chaos. So go ahead and grab a group together for book club or find colleagues who can meet up to play pickleball. Dust off your old camera to take pictures or tinker around with all the paints in your arts and crafts bin. Be sure to chat it up with your neighbor who is out gardening too. You can find me practicing for our next dance performance. By taking time out to make these things happen, we can squeeze in so much joy into our lives—and help make our worlds both in and out of medicine more enjoyable.

It may sound like too simple of a panacea—but the beauty with social prescribing is that we don't need a prescription pad at all. We just need to hit play.

Anita Bangale, MD, FACEP

Emergency Medicine Physician

President, Bangale Emergency Solutions

CEO and Founder, Diya Coaching

Physician Leader, Brightside Health

www.anitabangale.com

TEDxRaleigh Integrating Mental Health with the Power of Social Prescription—https://www.youtube.com/watch?v=9_az_wCrL4U

TEDxBreckenridge Masking Up in the ER to De-Armor and Connect—https://www.youtube.com/watch?v=PctYfeyWhc4

www.linkedin.com/in/anita-bangale-md/

Instagram @diyacoaching

References

Goebert D, Thompson D, Takeshita J, Beach C, Bryson P, Ephgrave K, et al. Depressive symptoms in medical students and residents: a multischool study. Acad Med. 2009;84(2):236–41.

Goldman ML, Shah RN, Bernstein CA. Depression and suicide among physician trainees: recommendations for a national response. JAMA Psychiatry. 2015;72(5):411–2.

Holt-Lunstad J, Smith TB, Layton JB. Social relationships and mortality risk: a meta-analytic review. PLoS Med. 2010;7(7):e1000316. https://doi.org/10.1371/journal.pmed.100031.

Khadilkar A. A conversation about suicide during medical training. JAMA Neurol. 2022;79(5):439–40.

Schwenk TL. Resident depression: the tip of a graduate medical education iceberg. JAMA. 2015;314(22):2357–8.

A Different Kind of Hero

42

Jillian Bybee

In 2020, during the initial surge of the COVID-19 pandemic in the United States, the general public began referring to those of us in healthcare as "heroes." It was a way of trying to recognize and thank us for the work that we were doing. A hero is someone who is admired or idealized for courage, outstanding achievements, or noble qualities. While this definition can easily be applied to healthcare workers who go above-and-beyond to help those in need, the message never seemed right to me.

To me, the use of the word *hero* in the context of the pandemic suggested that the public wanted a *superhero:* a benevolent being who fills the role of hero and also has *superhuman* abilities. This implies that healthcare workers do not have the same needs as others. And, as such, being a healthcare superhero leaves no room for humanity. As a younger person first entering the field of medicine, I believed in the myth of the "perfect doctor," and I tried to cover my own imperfections to fit. However, after personally experiencing struggles during medical training, I know that believing doctors are superhuman is one of the dangerous myths that we perpetuate. Since then, the "hero" story has not resonated with me. But a recent email from a colleague has challenged me to reassess my beliefs.

After I participated in a panel discussion for Physician Suicide Awareness Day, an email from a respected colleague appeared in my inbox entitled, *"You are such a hero to me."* It went on to talk about how my willingness to self-disclose about my experience with major depressive disorder during pediatric critical care medicine fellowship made them feel seen based on their experience with mental illness in their family. They thanked me for being willing to talk openly about issues that are often kept private. As I sat rereading the title a few times, I teared up, just as I had when I shared my story during the panel. I didn't feel much like a traditional hero, let alone a superhero. Instead, I felt vulnerable. But surprisingly, I also felt proud.

J. Bybee (✉)
Michigan State University, East Lansing, MI, USA
e-mail: jillian.bybee@helendevoschildrens.org

K. M. Schroeder (ed.), *The Essential Guide to Healthcare Professional Wellness*,
https://doi.org/10.1007/978-3-031-36484-6_42

At one point in my career, I may have felt shame for allowing myself to show emotion in public, but not anymore.

As someone who grew up in a family who didn't speak about emotions or our history of mental illness, learning to share has been a journey. At first, it seemed shameful. It took years to overcome my original programming and ignore the hidden curriculum of medical training which seeks to silence acknowledgement and sharing of difficulties. I began with first sharing privately in therapy and with those closest to me. This allowed me to begin to understand and process the secondary trauma and emotional devastation that comes from regularly witnessing serious illness and death. By hearing the stories of others, I came to realize that I was not alone and that my human emotions did not diminish my success as a physician. Along the way, my shame diminished because, as shame and vulnerability researcher Brene Brown says, *"Shame cannot survive being spoken. It cannot survive empathy."*

The psychologist Susan David speaks about emotions being signals and signposts for us. There are, she says, no negative or positive emotions. Rather, emotions give us data that we can, if we listen, interpret and respond to. In the best case, we do this skillfully, using the information as a way of understanding what is happening for us in the moment. In my case, I have spent most of my life doing this unskillfully (read: not acknowledging emotions at all). Fortunately, through therapy, learning, and connecting with colleagues, I found a better way.

My recovery from depression took years and remaining in remission takes ongoing work. It has taken becoming more in touch with my emotions, acknowledging my own humanity, and practicing self-compassion when I fall short of my own high expectations. I have had to allow myself to show up and be seen as a whole person with my own imperfections, not as the perfect superhero mythologized by my younger self and the medical field. This, according to Brene Brown, is one of the key aspects of courage because, as she often says, *"There is no courage without vulnerability."* And nothing is more vulnerable than choosing to let yourself be seen without knowing what the outcome will be.

Self-disclosure takes an immense amount of courage. I still feel somewhat afraid of being judged each time that I share because I never know how people will react. But the act of sharing has allowed me to connect with others, allowing them to seek help or share their own stories. I am motivated by my desire to normalize physician mental health struggles and to help others through my sharing. As I reflect on the definition of hero in the context of my own struggles, perhaps my colleague is right. I'm not a superhero without vulnerabilities. But I am, because of vulnerability and the courage required to tolerate it, a different kind of hero making an impact for others.

Jillian Bybee, MD, FAAP
She/her/hers
Assistant Professor
Section of Pediatric Critical Care Medicine at Helen DeVos Children's Hospital
Department of Pediatrics and Human Development at Michigan State University College of Human Medicine
Twitter and Instagram: @LifeandPICU
LinkedIn: www.linkedin.com/in/jillian-bybee-065335166

Prescriptions for Wellness

43

Kristopher Schroeder

As healthcare professionals, we are responsible for knowing all of the minutia associated with the care of our patients. We can easily recite the dosages and indications for scores of different therapeutics and can titrate these concoctions for the betterment of our patients. However, we occasionally suffer from awareness gaps in how to best care for ourselves and might benefit from a brief review of aspects of our life that we have evolved to ignore (potentially to our own detriment). Many of these aspects we know—I know I should not have ice cream while watching television before bed. Unfortunately, we suffer from a collective knowing-doing gap and gentle reassessments and reminders can be beneficial even for those of us that are approaching "well" or feel that there is no need for improvements. These basic considerations are important and taking care of ourselves will ensure that we are as "fit" as possible and better equipped to handle adversity and weather unpredictable wellness challenges.

For each of us, there are aspects of our wellness that might benefit from reappraisal and attention-based improvements. For example, sleep is critical for all humans and functions to clear brain metabolic waste products, modulate immune responses and metabolism, and improve energy conservation, cognition, performance, vigilance, and emotional wellbeing (Zielinski et al. 2016). Beyond benefits to the provider themselves, there is accumulating evidence that a lack of sufficient sleep can hamper the ability of healthcare professionals to provide compassionate and empathetic patient care (Gerace and Rigney 2020). Despite the important functions that sleep provides, we too often prioritize it below other functions or duties of far less perceived importance. Because of our chosen careers, some aspects and timing of sleep are truly beyond the scope of what we can control. If the only shift available to you is 2300-0700—there is not a lot that you are going to be able to do about the timing of your sleep. If you are on call and there is an emergency in the

K. Schroeder (✉)
University of Wisconsin School of Medicine and Public Health, Madison, WI, USA
e-mail: Kmschro1@wisc.edu

middle of the night, you can likely count on these types of sleep disturbances impacting your health and mental acuity for several days and the duration of the impact will likely increase as you age. Ultimately, if you focus on those aspects of sleep that are within your control there is a great opportunity to increase the quality/ quantity of your sleep and, through improved restfulness, positively impact multiple other facets of wellbeing. The American Academy of Sleep Medicine (AASM) as well as the CDC have several recommendations for better sleep (Sleep Education 2023; Tips for Better Sleep 2022):

Prescription for Better Sleep
- **Attempt to maintain a consistent sleep schedule**. Try to go to sleep and wake up at the same time every day (even when work is not on the agenda for the day)
- **Aim for 7–8 h of sleep per night**
- **Only go to bed when sleepy.** If unsuccessful with sleep efforts after 20 min, get out of bed and engage in an activity without significant light exposure
- **Adopt a relaxing routine prior to go to bed**
- **Use the bed only for sleep and sex**
- **Attempt to make the bedroom an oasis for sleep**. Keep it quiet, cool, and dark.
- **Limit exposure to bright lights, including electronics, in the evening**
- **Avoid large meals or fluid volumes before bedtime**
- **Avoid/limit alcohol and caffeine in the afternoon/evening**
- **Exercise regularly and maintain a healthy diet**

Exercise is another area of our lives that is too frequently neglected. Too often, we find that we lack the time required to get in a good sweat or that we are too exhausted at the end of the long day to even consider hoping on the treadmill. A survey of healthcare workers in Greece found that the top three factors limiting their ability to exercise were a lack of free time (58%), long work hours (41%), and pure negligence (37%) (Saridi et al. 2019). I know that in Wisconsin (we basically live beyond the wall—I apologize for the Game of Thrones reference), the idea of getting up before four o'clock to try and sneak in a run in the dark and the cold is a tremendous barrier to my January Walt Disney World marathon training. However, the payoff for making exercise a priority in our lives is huge and certainly more than worth the effort. Of course, one must weigh this early hour against the need for a full night of sleep.

Not only should we be physically active and exercise for our own well-being, but it also beneficially models behavior for our patients and families that can have long-lasting impacts. Our patients and kiddos are tremendous bullsh@#! detectors. If you are prescribing them an exercise regimen that you are not going to follow yourself, chances are not good that they are going to follow your advice and get moving. If you want to leave a legacy for your children, leave a legacy of loving physical activity. Leave a legacy of wanting to get out and hit the trails and enjoy nature. This is a gift that you can give to your children that they will hopefully pass on for generations. Beyond your patients and families, exercise in the workplace can have tremendous beneficial impacts for your colleagues as well. A study of Danish healthcare workers found that performing 10 minutes of exercise at work for 5 days per week resulted in an improved ability to handle the physical demands of the job and a decrease in absences due to sickness (Jakobsen et al. 2015). In an era of rampant staffing shortages, anything that improves the ability of the available workforce to be physically present and mentally well on a given day is certainly something worthy of administration consideration.

The benefits of a physically active lifestyle are immense and have the ability to impact a variety of health parameters. Physically active individuals are less likely to suffer from coronary heart disease, stroke, diabetes, bowel cancer, breast cancer, osteoarthritis, falls, depression, dementia, and early death (NHS 2022). Unfortunately, the default for many is physical inactivity. In fact, the World Health Organization reports that nearly one third of adults qualify as physically inactive and that 3.2 million deaths per year can be attributed to a lack of physical activity (World Health Organization 2022). The incidence of leisure time inactivity might be even worse in healthcare workers. A study of Brazilian healthcare workers found that leisure-time inactivity was 47.9% (Rocha et al. 2018). The immediate benefits of exercise are easy to see (improved health, sleep, mental health, physical function, etc.), but think about what you want your eventual retirement to look like. Don't you want to be the fun grandma/grandpa/aunt/uncle/friend that is still able to run around and keep up with the grandkids/nieces/nephews/peers? Don't you want to have the energy to travel and really enjoy the luxury of time? Exercise and a commitment to physical activity throughout your career will help you get to retirement in better shape and allow you to better enjoy that phase of your life. A steady commitment to exercise is routine maintenance for our bodies. Much like you wouldn't expect your car to get to 100,000 miles if you never changed the oil, we can't expect the same of our bodies. So what can we do to make ourselves and our physical fitness a priority?

Prescription for Incorporating Exercise Into Your Routine
- **Schedule exercise activities like you would any other commitment**. Make it so that exercise commitments occupy space on your calendar and that this is protected time.
- **Sign up for an event that is just outside of your current exercise comfort zone**. Push yourself a little if you can. If you are doing no exercise, sign up for a 5 k. If you are biking 10 miles, sign up for a 25 miler that gives you extra motivation to go out and do some additional training. If you are already doing Ironman events, God bless you, you can probably skip this section.

- **Turn meetings into opportunities for exercise**. For small meetings, why sit and stare at each other across a barren table? Moderate exercise stimulates the production of ideas and allows for the simultaneous accomplishment of exercise and productivity goals.
- **Turn your commute into an exercise opportunity**. If you can walk/run/ bike to work, that is outstanding and what an amazing opportunity to limit some time on your butt and simultaneously cut your carbon footprint.
- **Make exercise a social experience**. If you are lamenting not having enough time with your family, use exercise as a way to bring everyone together in group runs/bikes/etc. At work, consider the creation of monthly team competitions where the team with the most steps earns a coffee reward and bragging rights until the next round.
- **Have fun**. We have been given these amazing machines that allow us to do incredible things. What can you do to maximize the productivity of the machine that you have been given? How can you surprise yourself with the satisfaction associated with lifting a certain weight or covering a certain distance?

As we all know, the food that we choose to put into our bodies can have a profound impact on our health and wellbeing. Adopting a healthy diet can significantly impact the development of numerous cancers and also decrease the risk of cardiovascular disease. We know these things. I am not bothering to include a reference because these are things that we all know far too well as part of our zeitgeist. However, in our work environment, the adoption of healthy eating practices can be incredibly difficult. For one, in the course of our training we have frequently evolved to adopt a scavenger's mentality when it comes to food acquisition. Too often as trainees, did we take a chance on some breakroom delicacy of uncertain source or vintage. Stay overnight or even off-hours and the chances that the cafeteria is open get vanishingly small. This leaves healthcare workers desperate for sustenance left to sample the patients' supply of animal crackers and saltines or see what chips and candy bars are available in vending machines. When open, cafeteria offerings are frequently foods that seem more designed to result in hospitalization than improve nutrition or wellness. It is no surprise then that food delivery services to hospital settings represent a huge source of their daytime business. A study in China showed that Chinese physicians had placed over 170 million orders for take-out foods in only the first half of 2020 (Chen 2021). While these patterns develop during training, they can become entrenched and difficult to address when established in a career. Even now, the retirement of a colleague is a thing to be celebrated because we are at least treated to the cafeteria's finest cakes (the caring retirees will make certain to select our cafeteria's carrot cake offering). We all need to eat but the ideal diet depends on so many personal and health determinants that it is difficult to make sweeping recommendations without alienating some. However, there are some general principles that we can strive for.

Prescription for Improving Your Diet

- **If you can help it, don't get your food from the hospital**. Now, this doesn't mean that you should be ordering takeout for every meal either. But, if you can pack in a meal, it is most likely going to be better for you and cheaper than anything that you might be able to get at work. In addition, if you pack in food you will not have to wait in line at the cafeteria and it might afford you an opportunity to get in a short walk or other exercise, connect with a colleague, or complete some work project that you now will not have to take home.
- **Make it a family affair**. If you are going to pack in your food to work, use that prep time to simultaneously pack meals for your partner or children. This activity will ensure that the entire family unit benefits from your efforts to improve nutritional wellness and represents an easy way to gain some additional time together.
- **Limit the sweets**. This is tough—believe me, I know. Hospital wellness initiatives now frequently consist of some calorically dense morsel that is intended to demonstrate caring from on high. However, these empty calories are exactly what you do not need and, in many cases, may be responsible for many of the health issues that are plaguing our society. Stay away if you can. If you can't, cut the donut in half and leave the rest for some wayward scavenger later in the day.
- **Up your vegetable and fruit game**. Not always easy for everyone but experiment and explore all of the options out there to find something that works for you.
- **Drink some water and then drink some more**. Healthcare workers are chronically underhydrated. We do this to ourselves secondary to lack of time to drink and an unclear ability to use the restroom in the future. One of the highest risk work environments for underhydration is in in the operating rooms. In this environment, workers were shown to more regularly have decreased fluid intake and had nearly twice the risk of developing kidney stones. In the OR, 17.4% of physicians were found to have a history of kidney stones compare to 9.7% of non-OR physicians (Goldfarb 2016).

Overstating the negative potential consequences of alcohol consumption is difficult. Alcohol has been reported to cause 5% of the global disease burden and is responsible for 1:20 deaths (Albano et al. 2020). In the short term, alcohol consumption decreases inhibition, increases recklessness, impairs decision making, and decreases reaction time and coordination. While intoxicated, imbibers might suffer from an increased risk of accidents and injury, violence, unsafe sex, loss of possessions, and unplanned time off from work. If your intake of alcohol occurs when you happen to be working or on call, this could impact not only your ability to maintain employment but also the health of those whom you have sworn to care for. In high enough doses, alcohol consumption, by itself, can be lethal. These are only the short-term impacts of alcohol misuse. However, the unmentioned consequences (too loud karaoke, drunk dialing your ex, posting unflattering pictures to social media, and citations for public urination) are deeds that might also keep you up at night wondering what you were thinking. In the long term, multiple medical conditions (high blood pressure, stroke, pancreatitis, liver disease, cancers (liver, mouth, breast, bowel, head and neck), depression, dementia, sexual function disorders, and infertility can complicate wellness and introduce medical conditions with reaching impact. Alcohol abuse also significantly impacts those in your social sphere of influence. Because of the changes that occur in the setting of significant alcohol use and abuse, family break-ups, divorce, domestic abuse, unemployment, homelessness, and financial problems are burdens that, if you were drinking because of already existing problems, will not be made better through the use of alcohol. Despite the fact that we are flooded with commercials attempting to show us how alcohol intake will make our lives better, the reality is that significant alcohol intake is much more likely to make us end up alone and struggling with a collection of career/health struggles.

Having seen and cared for the adverse consequences of alcohol-related disease, we should collectively know better. However, it seems that there is something that compels our professions to seek comfort at the bottom of the bottle. Research has demonstrated that healthcare providers habitually consume alcohol at nearly two times the rate of the general population. In addition, nearly 1 in 5 healthcare workers consume alcohol at a rate that can be deemed either high or hazardous and that the risk of dangerous levels of alcohol consumption is increased in older women healthcare workers (Albano et al. 2020). If you are wondering if now is the time to cut down on your alcohol consumption, the truth is that it probably is. To better detect problematic drinking, John Ewing developed the CAGE Questionnaire as a mechanism to screen for problems with alcoholism (Ewing 1984).

CAGE Questionnaire
1. Do you sense that you should **C**ut down on your drinking?
2. Has criticism of your drinking from friends or family **A**nnoyed you?
3. Has drinking ever caused you to feel **G**uilty?
4. Do you start drinking early in the day or need an **E**ye-opener drink?

A score of 2 or more is considered to be clinically significant and should trigger efforts to reflect upon alcohol consumption and seek additional help if problematic drinking is detected.

Dry January has become a popular mechanism for our collective populace to "detox" from the holidays and adopt a healthier lifestyle with the changing of the calendar. If alcohol is a significant part of your life, waiting until an arbitrary astral location to initiate this change seems unwise. If the idea of a limited duration personal prohibition feels daunting, it is probably worth reflecting on the value of alcohol consumption and what it is providing versus what it is costing you. At some point, you may reach a point where health complications, relationship struggles, and inebriated entanglements will outweigh the benefits of intoxication. Hopefully, this realization occurs before there is a catastrophic incident with impaired driving or delivery of healthcare that forever stains your life.

Alcohol is not the only substance that we can elect to abuse that can negatively impact our health, relationships, well-being, and careers. A 2022 study evaluated the use of various substances in the ICU during the course of the COVID-19 pandemic and found that 11.2% of workers struggled with tobacco abuse, 24.7% with alcohol, 1.3% with cannabis, and 4.8% with hypnotics (Pestana et al. 2022). In certain careers, exposure and access to potent opioid analgesics makes these readily available and attractive drugs of abuse. Unfortunately, the ability to detect opioid abuse in our colleagues is limited and one of the first signs may be finding these colleagues either dead or unconscious in a bathroom. Even if these colleagues do find access to appropriate resources, data demonstrates that they are nowhere near to out of the woods. A 2015 study found that anesthesiology residents diagnosed with a substance abuse disorder had a significantly increased risk of mortality that persisted for 30 years following the initial diagnosis (Warner et al. 2015). The claws of these drugs pierce deeply and will forever impact those who choose to go down that path. At some point, you may find yourself approaching a branchpoint where you are considering ingesting or injecting an opioid or other anesthetic agent. Please, **do not**. Find help, talk to someone, or even take a leave of absence until you are able to reestablish a greater mental health foothold but don't go down this path.

For help with alcohol or substance abuse, there are abundant resources available. If one of these resources is not a good fit for you, don't stop, try another.

Alcoholics Anonymous (AA)	Secular Organizations for Sobriety (SOS)
www.aa.org	www.sossobriety.org
1-212-871-0974	1-323-693-1633
Centerstone	SMART Recovery
www.centerstone.org	www.smartrecovery.org
1-877-HOPE123	1-440-951-5357
Moderation Management	Substance Abuse and Mental Health Services
www.moderation.org	Administration
1-212-871-0974	www.findtreatment.samhsa.gov
National Institute on Alcohol Abuse and	1-800-662-HELP (4357)
Alcoholism	Women for Sobriety
www.niaaa.nih.gov	www.womenforsobriety.org
1-301-443-3860	1-215-536-8026

With regard to mental wellness, there are so many factors to consider that it is again difficult to offer a unifying prescription. Our careers have compelled us to engage in a number of behaviors that can diminish our mental wellbeing. Long hours of study and work may have eroded our social support network, constant fret over achievement may have fostered anxiety symptoms, previous adverse outcomes may result in PTSD, and a hostile work environment may serve as fertile ground for symptoms of depression. In some circumstances, witnessing and caring for victims of abuse, continuing to care for patients despite the futility of the circumstance, and abusive families can further contribute to a diminished sense of mental wellbeing. While escaping the demands of our profession may be difficult, there are certain habits that may alleviate some of the mental toll.

Prescription for Mental Wellness

- **Take your vacations.** We have evolved into a society that values business and work martyrdom far above wellness. As a badge of honor, we demonstrate our commitment to the profession by how many simultaneous tasks, meetings, and clinical days/shifts we can cram into a week. Vacation time is often the antidote to burnout and fatigue, but it has been reported that over half of the American public does not utilize their allotment of vacation time (U.S. Travel Association 2022). Take the time off that you have earned! You will come back from your vacation, whether you travel or not, more refreshed and productive.
- **Consider mindfulness activities.** How you achieve or approach these mindfulness activities, whether it is in a group/coached setting, through reading a book, or engaging with a podcast, may be less important than taking part in an exercise that allows you to acknowledge and accept your feelings and thought processes as legitimate. Use this time focusing on yourself to identify further areas for potential improvement and/or where additional help may be needed.
- **Get over worrying about how you might be perceived if you carry a diagnosis of depression, anxiety, or depression.** The reality is that you are not alone and the percentage of Americans with these diagnosis increases every year. With increased visibility, the stigma of these diagnoses diminishes, and the opinions of others is not worth the detrimental impact that inaction might have on your health.
- **Seek help**. Far too often, medical professionals suffer in silence from mental health disease that might otherwise be effectively treated. Please don't allow the perceived stigma of mental health disease prevent you from seeking the help that you need.

Finally, it is important to acknowledge that we are social creatures and that we are at our best and most resilient when surrounded by supportive family and colleagues.

Prescription for Social Wellness

- **Choose your influencers wisely**. It has been said that we are all an average of the five people with whom we spend the most time. Whether this idea is something that rings true or not, there is likely something to the idea of emotional contagion and how the negativity, or positivity, of others can impact our own mood or even actions. Given that you are most frequently able to choose who you spend your time with, make an effort to surround yourself with colleagues that exude positivity and happiness.

- **Be thoughtful in how you influence others**. If it is true that others have the ability to impact our own attitude and wellness, each of us may enjoy the blessing of influence over others. Use this power to try and lift up the attitude and wellness of your group and avoid giving in to negativity. At some point, uplifting the group may have a beneficial impact on your own situation.

- **Find a community**. You likely need people (I know that this is not true of everyone but playing the odds, most of you do). When you find your people, make sure that you treat them well and devote to them the attention and time that they deserve. These are hopefully the people that will be there for you at your low points and remain there when your career is nothing but a memory. As you work toward building this community of allies, don't restrict your applicant pool. A diverse supportive community (family, colleagues of diverse groups, friends outside of work) will help to reign in any siloed thinking that you might have and provide you with valuable perspective.

- **Serve**. Giving the valuable asset of time to another person or organization is a tremendous way to gain insight into those aspects of life that truly represent hardship. There is no better way to appreciate and elevate gratitude for what you have than to help those that have nothing.

- **Avoid falling into a social comparison pitfall**. At one point in our pasts, our small and isolated communities offered multiple opportunities to be recognized as the "best" in one area or another. However, our increasingly connected world has substantially limited the ability for us to really consider ourselves the "best" in any given area. Think that you are fast runner, there certainly is someone faster. Think that you are good looking, there is certainly someone that puts you to shame. Think that you had a great vacation, someone else travelled twice as far and for twice as long. Think your kids are great, well they certainly are not as great at "x" as one of your colleagues' kids. While the various social media platforms can offer great opportunities to learn, connect, and educate, there is a price to be paid for indulging in a world that frequently only shows everyone at their best. Exercise caution with these platforms as there is emerging evidence, especially in teens, that social media utilization can increase the risk of depression, anxiety, loneliness, and suicidal thoughts. The key in our increasingly connected world is to not be dismayed by the accomplishments of others. Instead, you should attempt to evaluate these posts knowing that they are only the brightest reflection of what is the reality of the poster. Try to simultaneously recognize and celebrate the accomplishments of the poster without undue comparisons to your own life or situation. While the social media poster may have just published their 800th paper in 2 years, you know nothing of their home situation or health. Even if they are rocking every aspect of life, their success should in no way impact your own and you should ensure that your use of social media does not cast a shadow over your own life and cause you to devalue what you have accomplished. If you get to the point where you have identified that social media utilization is causing you harm, cut the cord and evaluate what the impact of this change is on your life.

- **Reflect on activities that might be causing you harm**. Video gaming systems are absolutely amazing! I can still recall the jealousy that I had for my neighbor's Atari and that system had nowhere near the graphics or immersive qualities of today's gaming systems. However, the danger associated with the escapism provided by these gaming systems is that it provides too easy of a mechanism to avoid real life issues and negatively impact the ability to attend to work activities and sleep. The same can certainly be said for other non-productive activities such as social media scrolling and on-line shopping. At some point we all need to shop, but if you are finding that any of these activities is negatively impacting other aspects of your life it may be past time to consider re-evaluating the role and value that they are providing.

Like any prescription, you may need to, at various timepoints, have your prescription refilled or your dose increased. At the same time, there are always new and improved agents that emerge that should be considered. However, keeping in mind the basics of what might contribute to your wellness is an important step along the way to ensuring that you are able to achieve wellness in your career, your life, and your relationships with those that matter.

I truly hope that you have enjoyed this book and that it has provided you with, at the very least, some entertainment and an enhanced ability to share in the perspectives and experiences of your colleagues. Please, feel free to reach out at happyinhealthcareproject@gmail.com if you are interested in contributing to a future edition.

References

Albano L, Ferrara P, Serra F, et al. Alcohol consumption in a sample of Italian healthcare workers: a cross-sectional study. Arch Environ Occup Health. 2020;75(5):253–9.

Chen W. Dietary health of medical workers: who's taking care of it? Hepatobiliary Surg Nutr. 2021;10(2):232–4.

Ewing JA. Detecting alcoholism: the CAGE questionnaire. JAMA. 1984;252(14):1905–7.

Gerace A, Rigney G. Considering the relationship between sleep and empathy and compassion in mental health nurses: it's time. Int J Ment Health Nurs. 2020;29(5):1002–10.

Goldfarb DS. The exposome for kidney stones. Urolithiasis. 2016;44:3–7.

Jakobsen MD, Sundstrup E, Brandt M, et al. Physical exercise at the workplace prevents deterioration of work ability among healthcare workers: cluster randomized controlled trial. BMC Public Health. 2015;15:1174. https://doi.org/10.1186/s12889-015-2448-0.

NHS. 2022. https://www.nhs.uk/live-well/exercise/exercise-health-benefits/. Accessed 31 Oct 2022.

Pestana DVS, Raglione D, Dalfior Junior L, et al. Stress and substance abuse among workers during the COVID-19 pandemic in an intensive care unit: a cross-sectional study. PLoS One. 2022;17(2):e0263892. https://doi.org/10.1371/journal.pone.0263892.

Rocha SV, Barbosa AR, Araujo TM. Leisure-time physical inactivity among healthcare workers. Int J Occup Med Environ Health. 2018;31(3):251–60.

Saridi M, Filippopoulou T, Tzitzkos G, et al. Correlating physical activity and quality of life of healthcare workers. BMC Res Notes. 2019;12(1):208.

Sleep Education. 2023. www.sleepeducation.org/healthy-sleep/healthy-sleep-habits. Accessed 15 Aug 2022.

Tips for Better Sleep. 2022. www.cdc.gov/sleep/about_sleep/sleep_hygiene.html#:~:text=Be%20 consistent.,smart%20phones%2C%20from%20the%20bedroom. Accessed 15 Aug 2022.

U.S. Travel Association. 2022. www.ustravel.org/toolkit/time-and-vacation-usage. Accessed 31 Oct 2022.

Warner DO, Berge K, Sun H, et al. Risk and outcomes of substance abuse disorder among anesthesiology residents: a matched cohort analysis. Anesthesiology. 2015;123(4):929–36.

World Health Organization. Global Health Observatory Indicator Metadata Registry List. 2022. www.who.int/data/gho/indicatormetadata-registry/imr-details/3416. Accessed 31 Oct 2022.

Zielinski MR, McKenna JT, McCarley RW. Functions and mechanisms of sleep. AIMS Neurosci. 2016;3(1):67–104.

Index

© The Editor(s) (if applicable) and The Author(s), under exclusive license to Springer
Nature Switzerland AG 2023
K. M. Schroeder (ed.), *The Essential Guide to Healthcare Professional Wellness*,
https://doi.org/10.1007/978-3-031-36484-6

Printed in the United States
by Baker & Taylor Publisher Services